KNOCKIN

AT THE
GATE OF LIFE

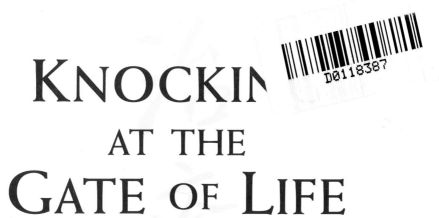

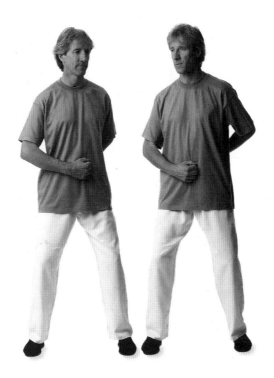

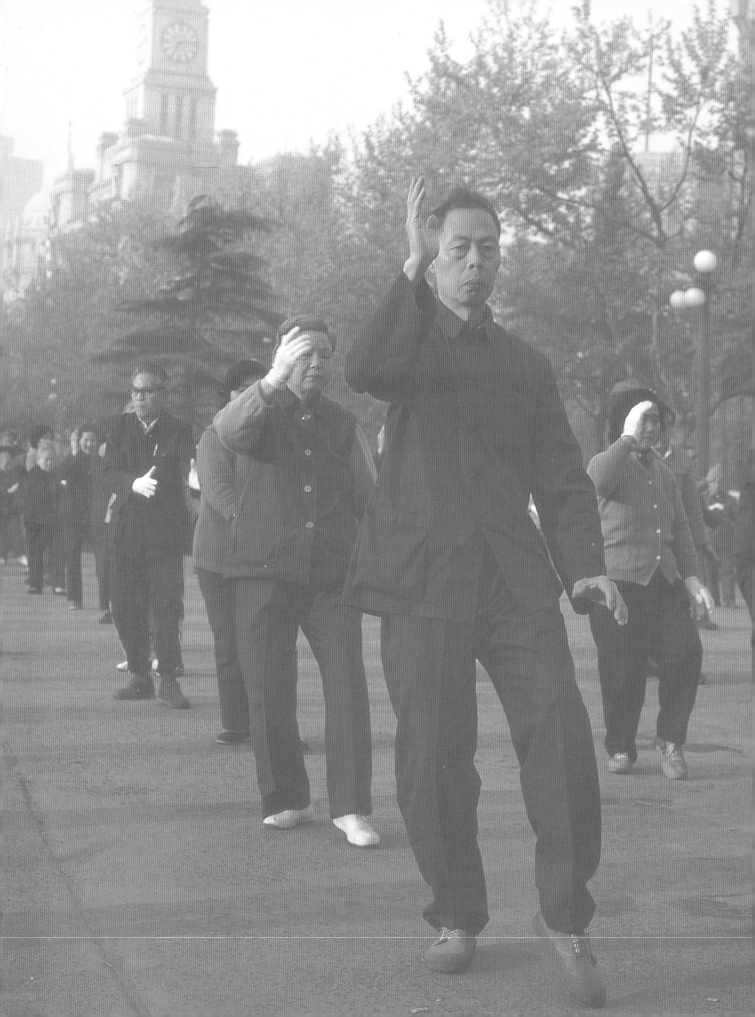

KNOCKING
AT THE
GATE OF LIFE

Healing Exercises from the

Official Manual of the People's

Republic of China

TRANSLATED BY

EDWARD C. CHANG

CONSULTANT EDITOR

PAUL BRECHER

LAUREL
GLEN

Published in the United States in 2000 by
Laurel Glen Publishing
An imprint of the Advantage Publishers Group
5880 Oberlin Drive, San Diego, CA 92121-4794
www.advantagebooksonline.com

Conceived, designed and produced by The Ivy Press Ltd
The Old Candlemakers, West Street, Lewes, East Sussex, BN7 2NZ.

ISBN 1-57145-662-7
Library of Congress Cataloging-in-Publication Data available upon request.

1 2 3 4 5   00 01 02 03 04

Creative Director: Peter Bridgewater
Designer: Kevin Knight
Publisher: Sophie Collins
Managing Editor: Anne Townley
Senior Project Editor: Rowan Davies
Consultant Editor: Paul Brecher @ Taiji.net
Editors: Lindsay McTeague, Mandy Greenfield
Studio Photography: Guy Ryecart
Illustrations: Andrew Kulman, Micheal Courtney
Three-dimensional Models: Mark Jamieson
Picture Research: Vanessa Fletcher

Typeset in Weiss and Gill Sans

Originated and printed in China by Hong Kong Graphic and Printing Ltd

Frontispiece: Early-morning Tai Chi exercises

North American Edition
Publisher: Allen Orso
Managing Editor: JoAnn Padgett
Project Editor: Elizabeth McNulty

Contents

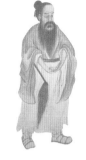
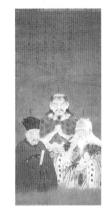
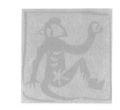

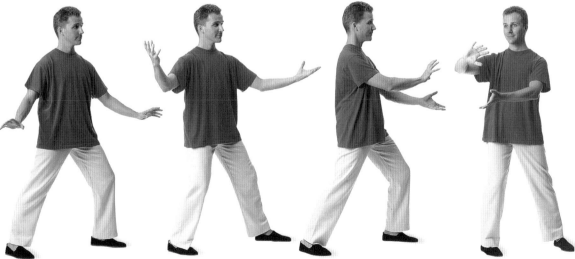

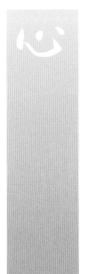

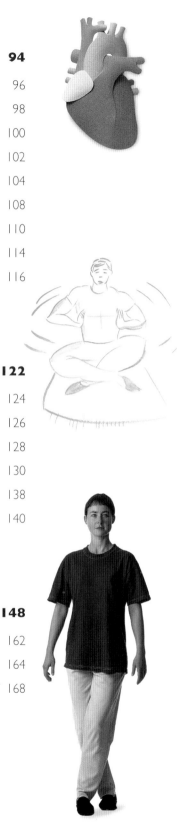

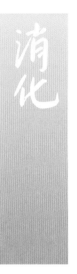

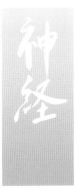

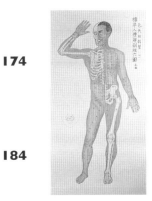

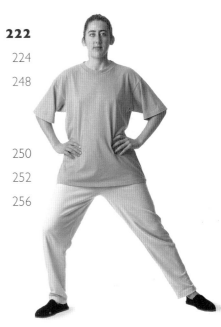

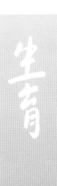

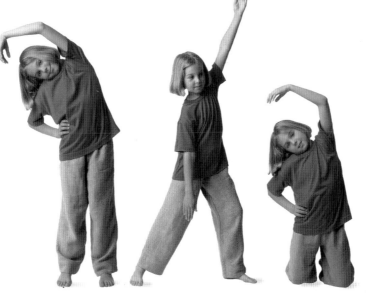

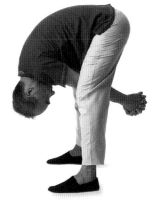

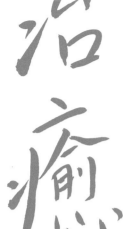

The Spiritual Background to Chinese Healing Exercises

If you are reading this book, the likelihood is that you are interested in leading a healthy life. You probably eat well, exercise regularly, and try to avoid activities such as smoking or excessive drinking that are likely to jeopardize your well-being. It may also indicate that you are interested in the wisdom that the ancient system of traditional Chinese medicine has to offer.

The first thing to recognize about the exercises in this book is that they actually have very little in common with aerobics, body-building, strength training, or any of the other exercise systems that are so common in the West. Masters of Tai Chi or Chi Kung—to name but two of the disciplines from which these exercises are drawn—are not concerned with building muscle or sculpting the perfect body. The real objective of these venerable Chinese systems is to build mental and physical well-being by encouraging the circulation of "chi" (*see p. 12*).

Traditional Chinese medicine says that each person is made up of three essential parts: mind, body, and spirit, or "shen." By performing the routines shown in this book you can begin to nourish all of these three elements at the same time. Practiced properly, these exercises can build self-confidence, boost your immune system, and give you a new sense of "balance" (a very important concept in traditional Chinese medicine—*see p. 13*) in your everyday life. As you will see, they can also help to relieve the symptoms of certain specific conditions; but as you practice each exercise, you should always consider the principles of balance, energy, and self-awareness that lie behind them.

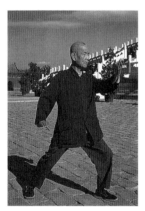

■ **Tai Chi being performed on the square in front of Beijing's Temple of Heaven.**

HOW TO USE THIS BOOK

The text is divided up into eight chapters, each of which deals with a different theme (*see pp. 5–7*). The first chapter (*see pp. 10–23*) contains essential information on traditional Chinese medicine (*see pp. 12–13*) and on the basic principles of healing exercise (*see pp. 14–15*), which you should read carefully before you begin doing the actual exercises themselves.

● The exercise spreads show all the steps of each exercise using photographs, with full explanatory text underneath.

● "Essential points" boxes draw out particularly significant information for the reader in a clear and succinct way.

● "Caution" boxes draw your attention to any health considerations which should be taken into account before the exercise is attempted, and you are advised to read these carefully.

● The diagrams of feet next to each photograph show you how your feet should be positioned and how your body weight should be distributed at each step.

● Introductory text provides background about the exercise and discusses any points of interest. Cross-references within the text show you where you can find related exercises and text in the rest of the book.

■ **Chi Kung breathing techniques are central to an understanding of the benefits of healing exercise.**

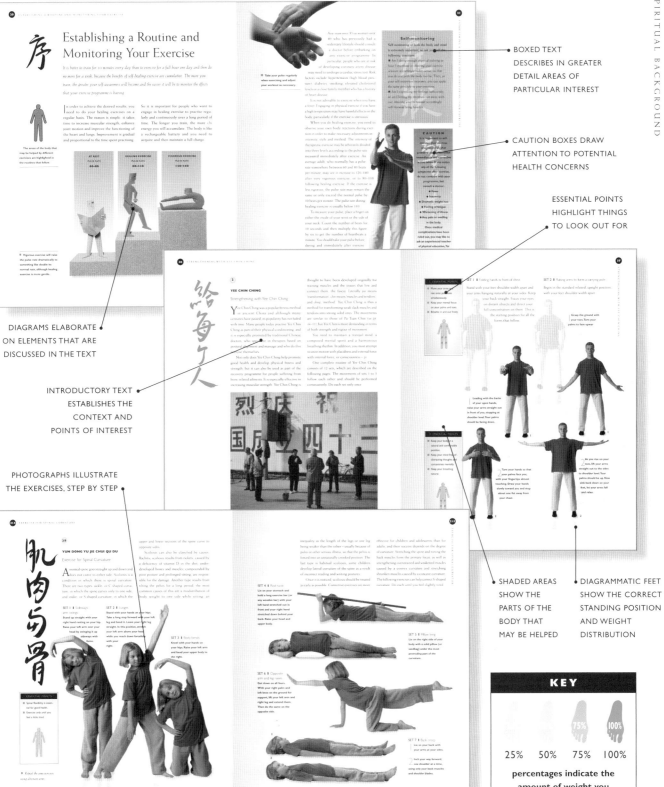

BOXED TEXT
DESCRIBES IN GREATER
DETAIL AREAS OF
PARTICULAR INTEREST

CAUTION BOXES DRAW
ATTENTION TO POTENTIAL
HEALTH CONCERNS

ESSENTIAL POINTS
HIGHLIGHT THINGS
TO LOOK OUT FOR

DIAGRAMS ELABORATE
ON ELEMENTS THAT ARE
DISCUSSED IN THE TEXT

INTRODUCTORY TEXT
ESTABLISHES THE
CONTEXT AND
POINTS OF INTEREST

PHOTOGRAPHS ILLUSTRATE
THE EXERCISES, STEP BY STEP

SHADED AREAS
SHOW THE
PARTS OF THE
BODY THAT
MAY BE HELPED

DIAGRAMMATIC FEET
SHOW THE CORRECT
STANDING POSITION
AND WEIGHT
DISTRIBUTION

KEY

25%   50%   75%   100%

percentages indicate the
amount of weight you
should put on each leg

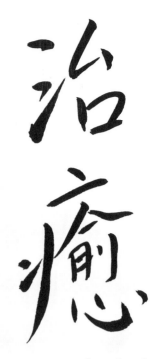

CHAPTER ONE

The modern world benefits from the self-healing systems of ancient China

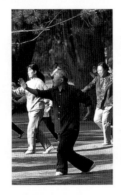

■ **Present-day Chinese use self-healing exercises in exactly the same way their predecessors did.**

Since ancient times there has been a philosophical system in China that underpins the healing arts, martial arts, and spirituality. The principles of the Tao, of Yin and Yang, *chi*, and the Five Elements form the framework for acupuncture, Chinese herbal medicine, martial arts, and Chi Kung (self-healing exercises, or The Art of Breathing). This book can provide only a brief overview and some simple introductory examples of easy-to-perform sequences to help heal a wide variety of ailments. The movements are taken from various famous Chi Kung and martial arts forms, which have been used in mainland China for hundreds of years with great success and are just as applicable today as they have always been. If you can attain a positive attitude and a calm and steady mind through the regular practice of Chi Kung, then you can heal the body and create a sense of well-being. Self-healing exercises balance the energy in the body by means of the meridians to enable you to regain good health, recover from injury, and improve the body's resistance to disease.

■ **The natural beauty of the Chinese landscape mirrors a belief in the power of inner calm.**

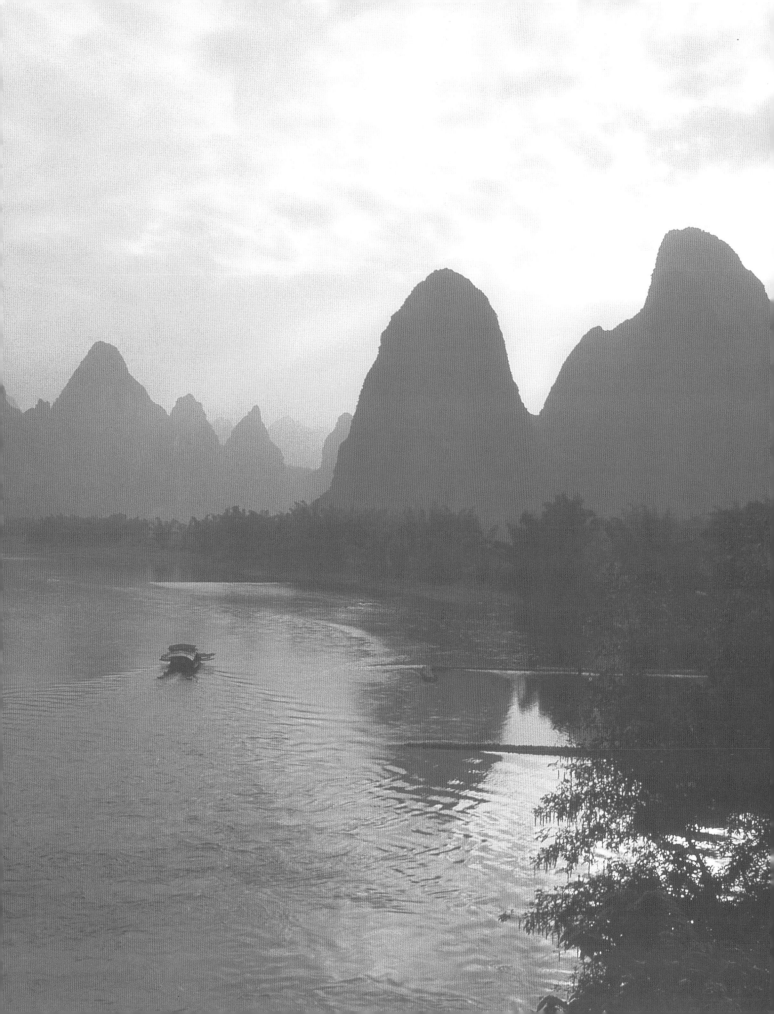

Healing Exercise and Traditional Chinese Medicine

The technique of Chi Kung has been practiced in China for over 6,000 years and it was the development of this Art of Breathing that led to discovery of the energy channels, or meridians, that run throughout the body, and from which the system of acupuncture was subsequently developed. Martial artists in turn then incorporated this knowledge into their own training.

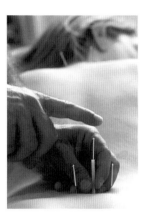

■ **Acupuncture points are located along the body's energy channels.**

In order for you to get the most out of the exercises that follow, you should first learn a little more about the basic principles of traditional Chinese medicine (TCM), which has been practiced in China for nearly 5,000 years. Many of the principles of TCM are also relevant to the Chinese martial arts which are shown in this book.

"CHI"

Chi is the universal life force, and it exists in the body in various forms. When our *chi* is in harmony, we enhance and preserve not just our health but also our capacity for fulfilment, happiness, and well-being. *Chi* is responsible for all the processes in the body and acts as a catalyst for metabolic change; it is also responsible for changes in our energy state, which affect our mind and spirit. Some people are born with good *chi*, but an unhealthy lifestyle will soon deplete their resources; other people may be born with sluggish *chi*, but they manage to boost it through careful stewardship. We all need to work at keeping our *chi* in top condition, and to ensure that there are no blockages which are preventing it from traveling freely throughout the body.

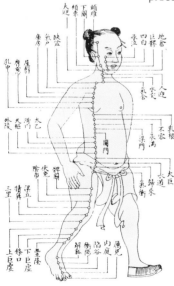

■ **Ancient Chinese tracts identified a wealth of acupuncture points on the body.**

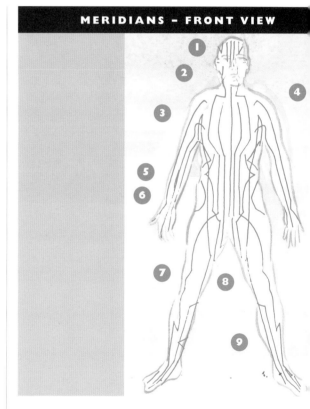

MERIDIANS — FRONT VIEW

MERIDIANS

Meridians are the energy channels or pathways along which *chi* flows to the organs and body parts. Most acupuncture points are sited along these channels, and most herbs prescribed by a physician will enter one or more of the meridian pathways. There are 12 main meridians, each corresponding to one of the 12 main organs of the body. There are also other minor meridians.

THE TWELVE ORGANS

Organs in TCM are categorized according to their perceived function, rather than their literal function as described by Western medicine. The 12 main organs according to TCM are the Lungs, Liver, Gall Bladder, Large Intestine, Bladder, Small Intestine, Spleen, Stomach, Kidneys, Heart, Pericardium, and an allegorical organ, the Triple Heater, which does not physically exist but which is believed to play a role in the movement of water around the body. Each organ has a designated meridian, and conditions which are believed to be caused by disharmonies within a particular

MERIDIANS – BACK VIEW

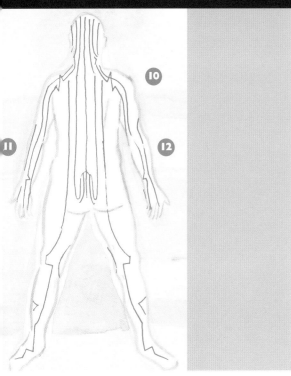

■ Each of the 12 main organs of the body relates to a specific meridian in traditional Chinese medicine.

organ will be treated by tending to the relevant meridian. For example, if someone has weak lungs, causing respiratory problems, then acupuncture points along the lung meridian will be needled in order to increase the *chi* energy (functional power) of the lungs.

YIN AND YANG

Yin-Yang is the way in which ancient Chinese philosophers made sense of the world around them. Essentially, it is a system of opposing forces and the pursuit of balance. It can be applied to all things around us including the workings of the human body.

The qualities that are associated with Yin are: coldness, darkness, dampness, calm, passivity, downward movement, supportiveness, and moisture; the qualities that are associated with Yang are: warmth, brightness, dryness, restlessness, activity, upward movement, and leadership. Nothing is totally Yin or totally Yang: all living things contain parts of both Yin and Yang, and the balance between the two forces will constantly shift.

Yin-Yang is also a comparative concept: a glass of lukewarm water will be Yang compared with an ice cube, but Yin compared with boiling water. When it is related to human health, Yin-Yang stresses the Chinese belief in the importance of balance; TCM practitioners will associate certain symptoms (dampness, coldness, listlessness) with an excess of Yin and will prescribe herbs or exercise to encourage Yang; in the same way, they will interpret heat, fever, dryness, and irritability as an excess of Yang and will try to encourage the presence of more Yin energy through their treatment.

As an example of the ebb and flow of Yin and Yang in the human body, we can look at what happens in the case of heatstroke. Extreme external heat (Yang) invades the body and becomes internal (Yin). This heat (Yang) burns off the body fluid (Yin), causing dehydration (deficiency Yin) and a high temperature (excessive Yang). So the patient is given Chinese herbal medicine in the form of a cup of tea. This contains cold (Yin) herbs to reduce the (Yang) heat, and nutritional (Yin) herbs to replenish the depleted body fluids. By this means Yin and Yang are brought into harmony once more and the patient makes a full recovery.

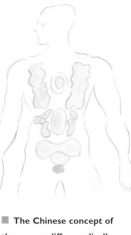

■ The Chinese concept of the organs differs radically from Western anatomy.

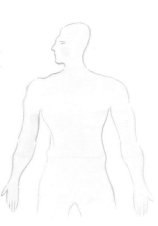

■ The Triple Heater, an allegorical organ which moves water around the body.

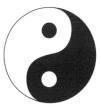

■ The Yin-Yang symbol shows that all Yin contains a little bit of Yang, and vice versa.

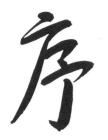

Healing Exercise Basics

If an individual practices self-healing exercise, this sends a positive message to the body's immune system, encouraging the body's healing mechanism to help itself, rather than rely on someone else (a health practitioner) to heal it. A passive attitude, on the other hand, sends a defeatist message to the body and will do nothing to stimulate self-healing.

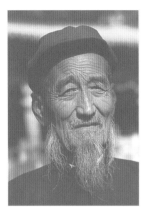

■ **The practice of healing exercise contributes to long life and good health among Chinese people.**

Wherever you go in China during the morning, you will see men and women doing healing exercises to protect or restore their health. But what exactly is healing exercise? It is simply exercise that has been shown to have significant therapeutic value. It can both treat and prevent certain diseases.

Healing exercise differs from regular exercise and other therapeutic techniques in several ways. First, healing exercise is designed primarily for— but is not necessarily limited to—people who are either sick or physically weak. It is used, for instance, to treat patients who suffer from chronic, or long-lasting, illnesses. The nature of the illness and the patient's condition and

habits determine the type of exercise to be used, and individual exercises may be modified in order to suit special needs, preferably under the guidance of a health professional.

Second, healing exercise does not rely on drugs, medicine, or surgery. Instead, it is designed to build up the patient's physical strength and improve his or her physiological functioning.

Third, healing exercise frequently involves the coordination of mind and body. That is why Chi Kung (The Art of Breathing) and Tai Chi Chuan (Yin-Yang Boxing) are especially effective in treating diseases that are closely linked to the emotions such as colitis, depression, hypertension, and peptic ulcers.

■ **In healing exercise, mental attitude is as important as the movements of the body.**

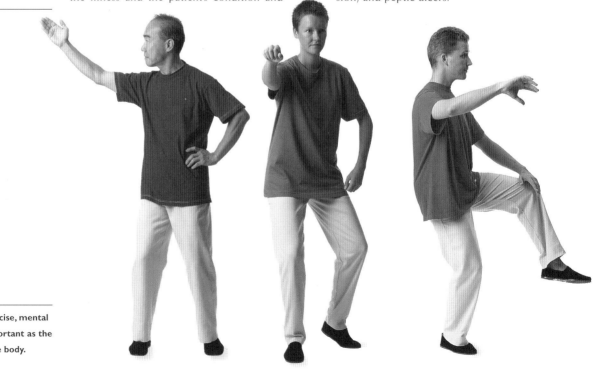

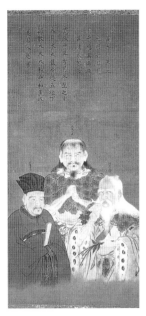

Huan Ti, Fu Hsi, and Chi'en Nung all played a significant role in Chinese medicine.

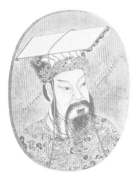

The Yellow Emperor, whose book, the *Neijing*, is a formative work on TCM.

THE DEVELOPMENT OF HEALING EXERCISE IN CHINA

Although the term "healing exercise" was only coined relatively recently, the use of physical exercise as a therapeutic technique can be traced back to about 1000 BC in China. The ancient Chinese probably accidentally discovered the value of massage and exercise in relieving pain and improving joint motion as they rubbed and pressed muscles that had become sore as a result of hard physical labor.

Even earlier—in the period of Tan Yao (2360 BC)—people used dancing as a form of therapy for arthritis. Later, during the Warring Period (403–221 BC), Dao Yin (psycho-physiological exercise) and Ta Na (breathing exercise) were introduced by the Taoists as effective techniques for the prevention and treatment of certain ailments. Archeologists working in Changsha recently unearthed artefacts including remnants of embroidered silk showing different postures used in meditation and exercise, which attest to the antiquity of therapeutic exercise in China.

Toward the end of the Han dynasty, a medical specialist named Hua To (AD 141–203) advocated physical exercise to improve resistance to disease. His system of healing is called Wu Chin Hsi (Five Animal Play). It imitates the movements of tigers, deer, bears, monkeys, and birds. Later, Tai Chi Chuan (Yin-Yang Boxing), Pa Tuan Chin (The Eight Sets of Embroidery), and Shih Erh Tuan Chin (The Twelve Sets of Embroidery) were invented and became popular. These exercises were found to be effective in preventing disease. Documents such as *Neijing* ("The Classic of Internal Medicine") and *Tsien Chin Fang* ("The Thousand Prescriptions") chronicle the history and methods of healing exercises.

5,000 YEARS OF HEALING EXERCISE

IN THE EAST	IN THE WEST
c. 2700 BC The art of silk weaving is mastered for the first time in China, together with the ability to make bronze items.	**c. 2600 BC** The epic of Gilgamesh relates how the Mesopotamian king tried to defy the gods in his search for immortality.
c. 1450 BC The city of Zhengzhou in China becomes the capital of the Shang dynasty.	**c. 1460 BC** An elaborate mortuary temple is built near Karnak in Egypt for Queen Hatshepsut.
c. 630 BC The *Book of Songs* is compiled, becoming *the* book to be seen with for educated Chinese.	**648 BC** Pankration, a combination of boxing and wrestling, makes its début at the Olympic Games.
AD 247 In Japan civil war breaks out as the dead queen's brother overthrows the female right of inheritance.	**AD 260** The Roman empire comes under attack from all sides: in the East, in Europe, and in Africa.
AD 477 Buddhism undergoes a revival and becomes the state religion in China, as Taoism begins to wane.	**c. AD 500** In Mexico the city of Teotihuacan becomes a huge political and religious capital of almost 250,000 inhabitants.

Why Healing Exercise?

The physical body, the mind, our energy, and spirit are all interconnected, but whereas the last three concepts are intangible and difficult to manipulate, the body is by comparison relatively easy to both understand and control. And by making the body stronger and healthier, we can influence the mind, energy, and spirit to become more balanced and whole.

Healing exercise helps to cure disease. Both repeated scientific experiments and patients who have actually used these exercises can testify to this.

Therapeutic exercise effectively prevents and treats diseases by correcting a number of problems. Some diseases stem from work habits. For instance, those people who have a sedentary job may have slack abdominal muscles and weakened intestines, with the result that they may be prone to chronic constipation. Others may develop neurasthenia, a common mental and physical condition which is characterized by lethargy, depression, fatigue, and sometimes insomnia, because of their concentration on mental activity without any form of physical exertion. Of course, a balance between mental and physical activities should be the goal that we try to achieve at all times.

Diseases triggered by weaknesses of the heart and lungs—emphysema and chronic circulatory problems, for example—can be helped by healing exercises. Both lungs and heart, respiratory and circulatory functions, may grow stronger.

In the treatment of diseases such as tuberculosis, high blood pressure, and diabetes, healing exercise can have secondary benefits. Although medication is needed when such diseases have reached a critical stage, if the patient's organs are too weak and their function too impaired, drug therapy alone may not be adequate. Regular healing exercise can strengthen the internal organs and increase the efficiency of the metabolic process, making it easier for the body to respond to the medication.

Some patients who suffer from chronic diseases have become so accustomed to a passive life that they have lost the desire to engage in almost any form of physical activity. As a result, the physiological function of their bodies tends to become weak. The effect of a lack of exercise over a prolonged period may show in symptoms such as depression, difficulty in breathing, circulatory problems, weak heart, problems with digestion, metabolic imbalance, muscle tightness, and even shrinkage of muscles. When this happens, the patient may be vulnerable to other diseases, as well as finding it difficult to recover from the original problem. But by doing exercises that will improve the performance of major internal organs, help regulate respiratory and blood circulation, and revitalize the digestive system, a patient can begin to regain lost health.

■ **A regular routine of physical exercise will always promote good health.**

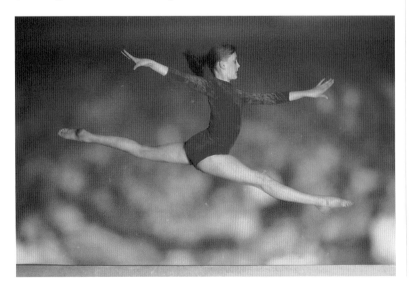

Some diseases are primarily related to the impairment of body movement, for example, immobility or stiffening of the joints or muscular paralysis. Tai Chi can improve joint mobility, strengthen nerves and muscles, and help a person to regain control of muscular movement. But all exercise has the benefit of increasing the flow of *chi*.

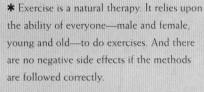

■ **Healing exercise can have a beneficial effect on the mind and spirit, as well as on the physical body.**

Benefits of healing exercise

The advantages of healing exercise are numerous. For one, it is easy to do. It is also cost-free, because it involves no special facilities, and its therapeutic effects are obvious. Some of the benefits of doing therapeutic exercise on a regular and systematic basis are as follows:

✱ Therapeutic exercise helps promote proper functioning of the heart, lungs, and joints. It also promotes muscular development, which cannot be achieved by the use of medicinal drugs.

✱ Healing exercise is a holistic therapy. Unlike other therapies that focus only on the affected part, exercise treats the entire body by toning the nervous system and the circulation of the blood. It also improves the body's ability to absorb and transport nutrients, thereby increasing immunity.

✱ Healing exercise is a form of self-therapy. The patient must actively participate in the treatment process and is therefore more inclined to develop a positive attitude toward the treatment, as well as greater confidence in his or her own power to affect the outcome. All of this can hasten recovery.

NERVOUS SYSTEM

LUNGS

HEART

BLOOD CIRCULATION

MUSCULAR DEVELOPMENT

JOINTS

✱ Exercise is a natural therapy. It relies upon the ability of everyone—male and female, young and old—to do exercises. And there are no negative side effects if the methods are followed correctly.

✱ Healing exercise is a preventive technique, and prevention, of course, is always better than cure. If you can improve your physical strength and increase your body's ability to resist diseases, then you may be less susceptible to sickness in spite of external factors. It is a fact that in similar circumstances some people get sick easily, while others remain healthy. This is because the healthy people have acquired the ability to resist the invasion of disease-producing agents by taking care of their internal health.

■ **As a holistic therapy, healing exercise is beneficial for both body and mind.**

Forms and Methods of Healing Exercise

The type of healing exercise that you should practice depends on your physical condition, your age, and your natural inclination toward certain activities. The six categories that are described here all form part of the Old Yang Style of Tai Chi Chuan, so this form of exercise is recommended more than any other system throughout this book.

Healing exercise may be divided into the six categories of therapeutic gymnastics, exercise therapy, mechanical therapy, Chi Kung (The Art of Breathing), An Mu (massage), and recreational exercise.

※ **Therapeutic gymnastics:** Of all the types of healing exercises, therapeutic gymnastics deserve special attention because of their effectiveness. Each exercise has a purpose and is specially chosen to help heal specific diseases. For example, the therapeutic gymnastics for chronic bronchitis probably differ from that which are intended for relieving pain in the waist and leg, just as exercises for high blood pressure are quite unlike those that are used for treating emphysema.

A therapeutic gymnastics session will usually consist of between 5 and 20 series of exercises. Each series calls for special preparation, posture, exercise content, and number of repetitions. Emphasis, however, is placed on the quality of the exercise rather than on the amount or variety of it. Sometimes the same healing results can be achieved by means of a limited number of repetitions of the most effective exercises.

※ **Exercise therapy:** This type of exercise can help prevent and treat certain illnesses. It includes Tai Chi Chuan, various gymnastic exercises, walking, hiking, canoeing, taking field trips into the countryside, and other less rigorous sports. Generally speaking, exercise therapy is more effective than therapeutic gymnastics in improving the function of the heart and lungs. It is most appropriate for patients who are suffering from chronic illnesses, if they have the physical strength necessary to attempt them.

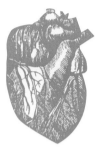

■ To have a positive effect on the heart, exercise should raise the rate at which it beats.

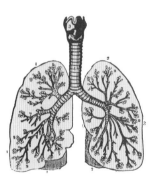

■ Much exercise is aerobic, which increases the intake of oxygen into the lungs.

■ It is all too easy to practice a sedentary lifestyle at work and fail to fit exercise into your daily routine.

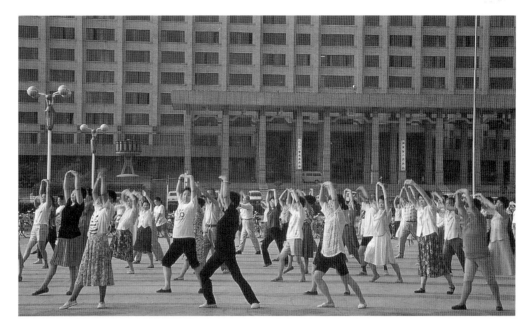

In China many people participate in collective exercises done in a city square or park before work.

❋ **Mechanical therapy:** This method calls for special exercise equipment. Its aim is to restore the normal function of the limbs and joints, and to help correct any deformities. An exercise bicycle, for example, can help strengthen leg muscles, while a specially constructed wheel can enhance the function of shoulder joints.

❋ **Chi Kung:** Mental concentration is combined with breathing exercises in Chi Kung. It is designed to cultivate and nourish *chi*, or energy flow, within the body. The Chinese have found that Chi Kung is an effective healer of many chronic diseases, including depression, high blood pressure, peptic ulcers, and duodenitis (inflammation of a portion of the small intestine).

❋ **An Mu:** Performed either by the patient or by a health professional, An Mu (massage) can ease pain, stimulate blood and lymphatic circulation, increase muscle flexibility, accelerate digestion, reduce fatigue, and relax muscles.

❋ **Recreational exercise:** Activities such as gardening, knitting, and other do-it-yourself hobbies can not only develop muscles but also relax the nervous system. They are an excellent way to encourage a sufficiently great amount of physical activity to help promote physical and psychological fitness.

This book deals primarily with exercise therapy and Chi Kung, but no healing exercise or physical therapy can be considered a panacea. Like any other therapeutic technique, each has limitations. One may be particularly useful for certain ailments, but have only minimal or secondary effects on others. Chinese doctors have found healing exercise most effective for treating the following types of diseases:

● Chronic diseases that are associated with the respiratory, digestive, cardiovascular, and reproductive systems.

● Paralysis that results from nerve injury or that is caused by impaired blood flow through the cerebral vessels.

● Stiff joints due to external injury or arthritis.

● Abnormal posture, such as curvature of the spine, or other structural problems to some degree—even flat-foot can be helped, if the case in question is not too severe.

● Depression and melancholia.

Establishing a Routine and Monitoring Your Exercise

It is better to train for 10 minutes every day than to exercise for a full hour one day and then do no more for a week, because the benefits of self-healing exercise are cumulative. The more you train, the greater your self-awareness will become and the easier it will be to monitor the effects that your exercise program is having.

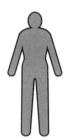

■ The areas of the body that may be helped by different exercises are highlighted in the routines that follow.

In order to achieve the desired results, you need to do your healing exercises on a regular basis. The reason is simple: it takes time to increase muscular strength, enhance joint motion, and improve the functioning of the heart and lungs. Improvement is gradual and proportional to the time spent practicing.

So it is important for people who want to engage in healing exercise to practice regularly and continuously over a long period of time. The longer you train, the more *chi* energy you will accumulate. The body is like a rechargeable battery and you need to acquire and then maintain a full charge.

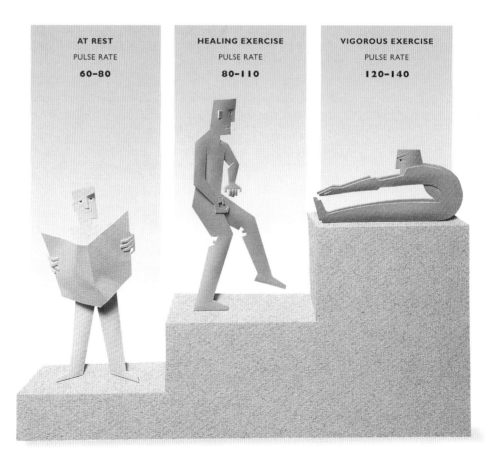

AT REST	HEALING EXERCISE	VIGOROUS EXERCISE
PULSE RATE	PULSE RATE	PULSE RATE
60–80	80–110	120–140

■ Vigorous exercise will raise the pulse rate dramatically to something like double its normal rate, although healing exercise is more gentle.

Take your pulse regularly when exercising and adjust your workout as necessary.

Any man over 35 or woman over 40 who has previously had a sedentary lifestyle should consult a doctor before embarking on any exercise program. In particular, people who are at risk of developing coronary artery disease may need to undergo a cardiac stress test. Risk factors include hypertension (high blood pressure), diabetes, smoking, elevated cholesterol levels, or a close family member who has a history of heart disease.

It is not advisable to exercise when you have a fever. Engaging in physical exercise if you have a high temperature may have harmful effects on the body, particularly if the exercise is strenuous.

When you do healing exercise, you need to observe your own body reactions during exertion in order to make necessary adjustments in intensity, style, and method. The intensity of therapeutic exercise may be arbitrarily divided into three levels according to the pulse rate measured immediately after exercise. An average adult, who normally has a pulse rate somewhere between 60 and 80 beats per minute, may see it increase to 120–140 after very vigorous exercise, or to 80–110 following healing exercise. If the exercise is less rigorous, the pulse rate may remain the same or only exceed the normal pulse by 10 beats per minute. The pulse rate during healing exercise is usually below 110.

To measure your pulse, place a finger on either the inside of your wrist or the side of your neck. Count the number of beats for 10 seconds and then multiply this figure by six to get the number of heartbeats a minute. You should take your pulse before, during, and immediately after exercise and adjust your workout if necessary, so that you are not overstraining yourself.

Exercise ranges from fast aerobic routines to more gentle, stretching movements.

Self-monitoring

Self-monitoring of both the body and mind is extremely important, so ask yourself the following questions:

* Am I doing enough physical training or have I overdone it? Altering your exercise sessions accordingly makes sense, so that you do not push the body too far. Then, as your self-awareness increases, you can apply the same principle to your emotions.

* Am I expressing my feelings sufficiently, or am I letting my emotions run away with me? Altering your behavior accordingly will likewise bring benefits.

CAUTION

It is important to self-monitor your exercise program so that problems can be identified immediately and corrective action taken. If you notice any of the following symptoms after exercise, do not continue with your program, but consult a physician:

● Fever
● Insomnia
● Dramatic weight loss
● Feeling of fatigue
● Worsening of illness
● Any pain or swelling in the body.

Once medical complications have been ruled out, you may like to ask an experienced teacher of physical education, Tai Chi, or Chi Kung to help you determine the cause— you may be doing the exercises incorrectly.

More Ways to Help Yourself Heal

Exercise should not be viewed in isolation, as the only way to help yourself heal. In fact, it should always be combined with a sensible diet and a practical approach toward the value of medication. Sleep is another important factor and, when all these factors are successfully combined, you stand the greatest chance of boosting your health.

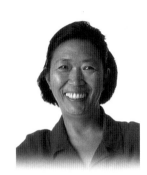

■ **Good health comes about through a combination of exercise, diet, rest, and play.**

Therapeutic exercise improves physical strength, helps the body to build up immunity, and enables it to combat existing disease. But although some chronic patients understand the healing value of exercise, they pay less attention to other important health factors such as eating, sleeping, and the psychological aspects of living. First of all, they should develop an optimistic spirit when it comes to combating disease. Patients who anticipate fighting a losing battle may be too worried to achieve any significant results even if they do exercise.

Those who are sick should work on a correct attitude toward medication. On the one hand, some patients have too much faith in therapeutic exercise and reject medicine. On the other, some may rely on medicine so much that they fail to see the value of other techniques. Both extremes should be avoided.

Medication may be necessary for treating both acute and chronic diseases during the development stage, and particularly later on, even though patients do healing exercise. Medicine may be reduced or discontinued only after the problem has been relieved as a result of regular exercise.

Those who are ill should pay special attention to the kinds of food and drink they consume. Good nutrition comes from eating a variety of foods, and it need not cost a lot. The most important thing is to have a balanced diet. Half of your daily food intake should consist of carbohydrates such as noodles, pasta, and rice. You should also eat at least five portions of vegetables and fruit a day. Proteins, including meat, fish, nuts, and dairy products, should be eaten in moderation, while consumption of sugar and fats should be strictly limited. Within these basic food groups, try to vary your selection so that you obtain all the essential nutrients.

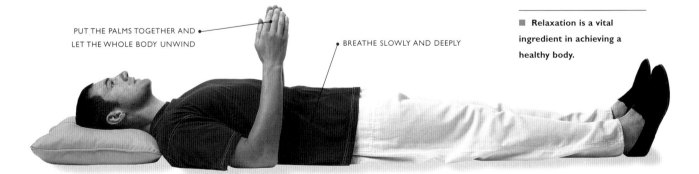

PUT THE PALMS TOGETHER AND LET THE WHOLE BODY UNWIND

BREATHE SLOWLY AND DEEPLY

■ **Relaxation is a vital ingredient in achieving a healthy body.**

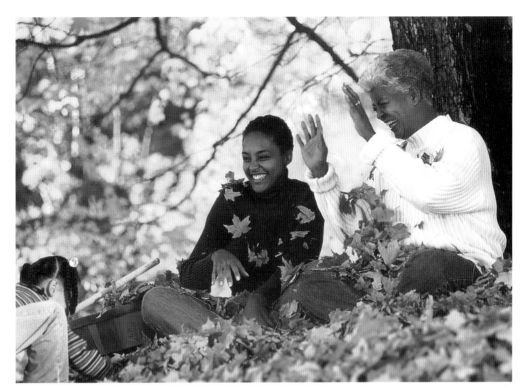

■ **It is just as important to enjoy your free time as it is to eat and sleep well.**

Patients should also keep a good balance between work and recreation, should set aside a particular time for exercise, and should adhere to a regular bedtime—if at all possible, it is most beneficial to sleep between 11.30pm and 7am, when the body is best attuned to making the repairs that take place during the hours of sleep, when the activity hormones shut down and the repair and maintenance hormones take over. In short, follow a regular routine.

Those with chronic diseases must stop smoking and drinking alcohol, since both of these activities have been found to impede the treatment of disease. Tobacco and alcohol produce toxins in the body, which in turn puts extra stress on the liver at a time when the body is already under considerable strain.

Patients who avoid smoking and alcohol and who follow a regular exercise program are those who will benefit the most from physical exercise therapy.

A healthy diet

Many people are aware of what constitutes a healthy diet, but find it difficult to put into practice. A lot of the essential nutrients that we need can be found in an abundance of fresh fruit and vegetables, so the maxim of five portions a day makes enormous sense. Ideally, food should be appropriate to the season, with fewer salads, ice cream, and cold foods in winter and more fruit in summer. But the main thing is to attain a healthy balance.

■ **A variety of fresh fruits, vegetables, and legumes, plus a little protein is ideal.**

CHAPTER TWO

Healing exercise can give you the strength of a bear, the agility of a deer

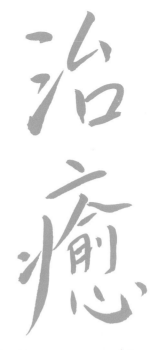

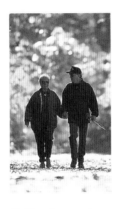

■ **Almost no one is too old or too young to benefit from healing exercise.**

Whether you are aged 9 or 90, a weight-lifter or too weak even to lift your arm, there are Chinese healing exercises for you. There are exercises that will make you feel more alive and vibrant when you wake up in the morning, and exercises that will soothe you and help you sleep better at night. Although primarily designed to strengthen and build resistance in people who are healthy, many of the exercises in this chapter can also help those suffering from nagging chronic diseases.

Some of the exercises, such as the ones known as The Twelve Sets of Embroidery or Five Animal Play, have been treasured, practiced, and polished over centuries and have a long history of healing. Others are more modern, but no less cherished and effective. With regular practice Five Animal Play, for instance, can help you develop the strong bones of a tiger, the strength of a bear, the agility of a deer, the flexibility of a monkey, and the grace of a bird. What is more, the benefits of such exercises are available to anyone who trains every day.

■ **Greater vitality and alertness are just two of the benefits of healing exercise.**

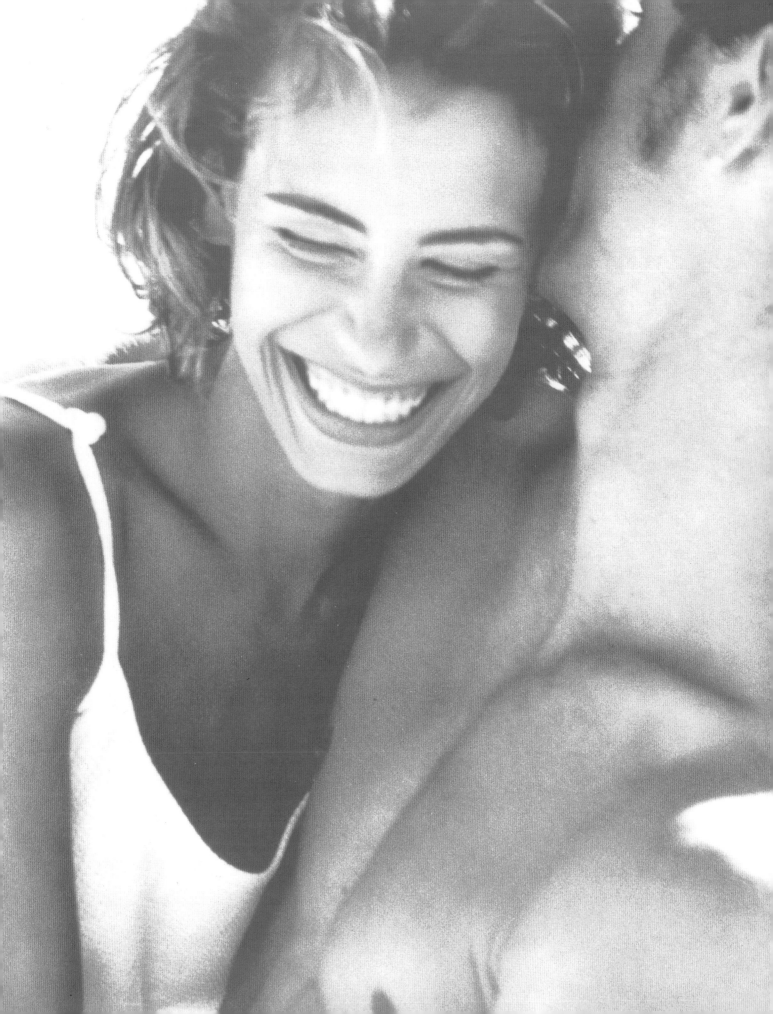

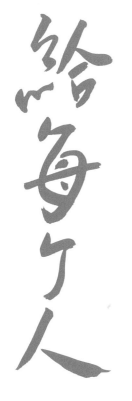

■ This Chinese calligraphy reads "healing exercise for everyone."

① WU CHIN HSI

Five Animal Play

Developed by Hua To, a famous Chinese doctor of the late Han dynasty, Wu Chin Hsi consists of movements that mimic the gestures and mannerisms of five different animals—a fierce tiger, a graceful-necked deer, a lumbering bear, an agile monkey, and a flying bird. For his time, Hua To was pragmatic and empirical in his approach to medicine. He was against superstition and attacked the traditional Confucianism-orientated medical theory built on supernaturalism. His Five Animal Play was based on his belief that exercise and medicine could be integrated in developing physical fitness and preventing and fighting disease. He developed his exercises more than a thousand years before the same idea was conceived in Sweden.

Many variations of the Five Animal Play have been added since Hua To's time; the original movements have been continuously modified and improved. The version on the following pages is easy to learn and is known to have good results. You may practice the whole set or choose part of it, depending on your needs.

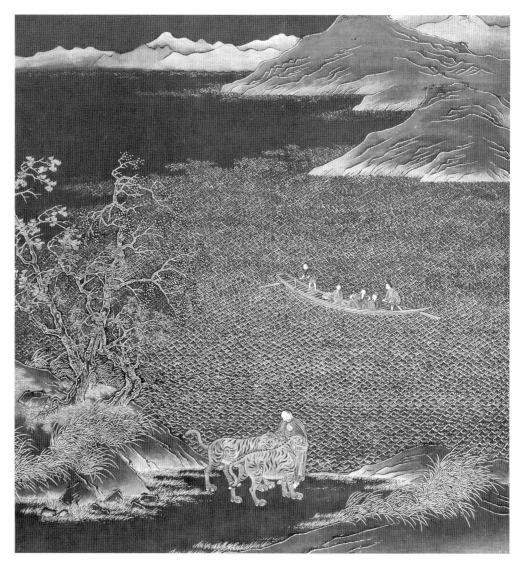

■ Five Animal Play is based on observation of the movement of Chinese animals in their natural habitat.

ESSENTIAL POINTS

- Be natural as you twist your waist and sway your groin.
- Be gentle as you relax and move your joints.
- Be graceful and steady as you set your feet on the ground.
- Be calm and focus your attention on Tan Tien (Field of the Elixir), an energy center about 3in (7.5cm) below the navel, from which *chi* can be directed to all parts of the body.

SET I ▍ Bear play

While you are performing this exercise imagine that you are a great big, powerful bear moving in a relaxed, natural way so that your whole body feels loose, heavy, and sturdy, and your arms hang naturally.

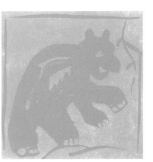

1 **Stand with your feet shoulder-width apart and your arms hanging loose and naturally. Breathe in and out deeply 3 to 5 times. Then sway your waist, your hips, and your groin in a natural but bearlike way.**

2 **Bend your right knee slightly and swing your right shoulder downward to the front with your arm hanging naturally. At the same time, turn your left shoulder slightly backward and lift your left hand slightly.**

3 **Reverse the position in step 2. Bend your left knee and swing your left shoulder down to the front with your arm hanging naturally, and turn your right shoulder slightly backward, lifting your right hand slightly.**

● *Repeat this exercise as many times as you like. It improves digestion, joint mobility, and the functioning of both the spleen and the stomach.*

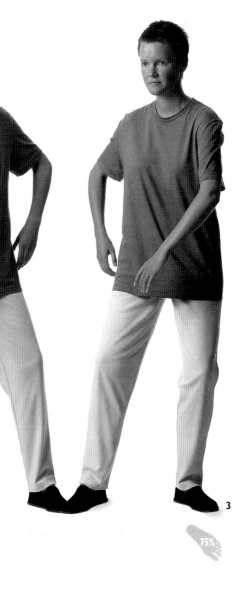

1

2

3

SET 2 | Tiger play

The making of the tiger-claw shape with the hands forms the main part of this exercise. As you perform this action, pull your hands down and toward you slightly, with the areas known as the "tigers' mouths" tightly stretched.

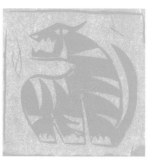

1 **Let your arms hang down naturally. Keep your neck straight and your face relaxed. Look straight ahead. Keep your mouth closed with your tongue gently touching the roof of your mouth. (The tongue should touch the roof of your mouth in order to connect the Governing Meridian with the Conception Meridian, allowing** *chi* **to flow through the body.) Do not bow or thrust your chest forward. Move your heels together to form a 90-degree angle. This is basically a standing-to-attention posture, but your whole body should be relaxed. Stand in this position for a few moments.**

2 **Slowly bend your knees to lower your body. With your weight on your right leg, lift your left heel slightly off the ground and bring it close to your right ankle. At the same time, form fists and bring them to the sides of your waist with the fingers facing up. Turn your eyes toward the left.**

ESSENTIAL POINTS

- Try to capture the fighting spirit of a tiger.
- Try to imitate the tiger's speed and grace.
- Be composed yet fierce.

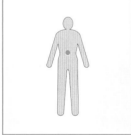

HANDS MAKE THE SHAPE
OF TIGERS' CLAWS

3 Then take one step forward to the left. Keep your right foot half a step behind. The distance between your heels should be about 12in (30cm). Keep your weight on your right foot and lift your fists toward your chest with the fingers facing your body. As your fists approach the level of your mouth, turn your fists over, open your hands and push out strongly at chest level with your palms open. Your so-called tigers' mouths—the space between your thumbs and index fingers—will be facing each other and should be tightly stretched. Their purpose is to activate the acupuncture point Large Intestine 4. Look at the tip of your left index finger with both eyes.

WEIGHT IS ON THE RIGHT FOOT

LEFT FOOT HALF A STEP IN FRONT

3

REPEAT THE EXERCISE

4 Repeat the sequence to the right. Starting again from the at-attention position, bend your knees, put your weight on your left leg, lift your right heel off the ground, and bring it close to your left ankle. Continue with the rest of step 2 and step 3 except that your direction is to the right. You can repeat the sequence as many times as you like.

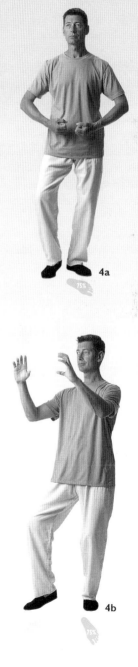

4a

4b

SET 3 ∥ Monkey play

To get the most from this exercise you need to synchronize the movements of the elbow and knee and of the hand and foot, so that the whole of your body moves fluidly together as a single unit. Stand to attention but relaxed for a few minutes, as for tiger play (*see pp. 28–29, step 1*).

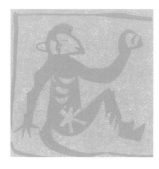

1 **Bend your knees slowly to lower your body. Step forward gracefully with your left foot. At the same time, raise your left hand up beside your chest. As soon as it reaches the level of your mouth, make it into a claw and thrust it forward as if you were reaching out to grasp an object.**

2 **Then step forward with your right foot and lift your left heel slightly off the ground. At the same time raise your right hand up beside your chest. When your hand is level with your mouth, thrust it forward in a clawlike position with your wrist bent. Bring your left hand back to your side with the elbow bent.**

3 **Move your left foot behind you and place it firmly on the ground. Bend that knee and shift your weight onto that leg. Move your right foot back slightly too, and lift your heel while keeping your toes on the ground. At the same time, raise your left hand. When it is level with your mouth, thrust it forward in a claw and draw your right hand back to your side.**

ESSENTIAL POINTS

- Try to coordinate your hand and feet movements in a smooth, continuous motion.
- Whichever foot your weight is on, the corresponding hand should be forward.
- Move gracefully and quickly.

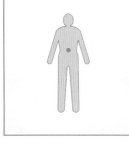

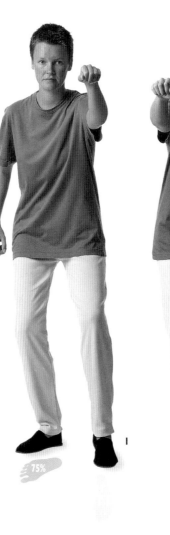

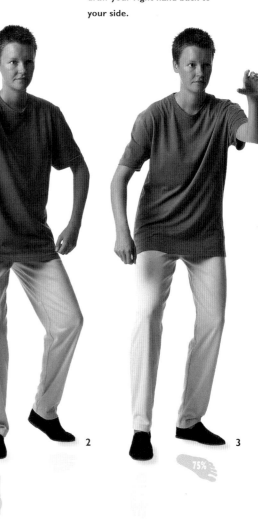

1

2

3

RIGHT HAND MAKES
A CLAW SHAPE LEVEL
WITH THE MOUTH

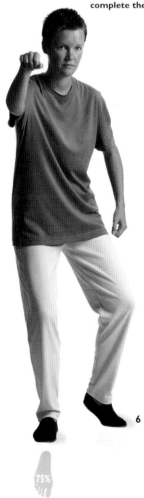

4 Quickly and gracefully, take one step forward with your right foot as you bring your right hand up in front of your chest. **Make a claw and extend it in a grasping motion as soon as it is level with your mouth.**

5 Step forward smartly with your left foot and follow with the right foot. **Lift your right heel while keeping your toes on the ground. At the same time, bring your left hand up to your chest. As soon as it reaches mouth level, thrust it forward in a clawlike shape. Draw your right hand back to your side with the elbow bent.**

6 Step back slightly with your right foot and place it firmly on the ground. **Bend your knee and shift your weight onto that leg. Move your left leg back slightly also. Lift that heel and keep your toes down. At the same time, bring your right hand up to your chest. As soon as it reaches mouth level, thrust it forward in a claw. Draw your left hand back to your side with the elbow bent to complete the exercise.**

4

5

6

75%

75%

SET 4 | Deer play

The ability of the deer to leap and bound gracefully is due to the agility and power of its hips. You too can get a spring in your step by practicing the Deer-play exercise in order to strengthen the area of the tailbone.

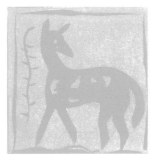

LEFT PALM FACES TO THE RIGHT

Bend your right knee and draw your upper body back. Extend your left leg forward with your knee slightly bent, keeping your weight on your right leg.

ESSENTIAL POINTS

■ This exercise is based on the notion that the deer frequently shakes its tail. If you rotate your arms—representing the deer's neck—in a larger circle, then your coccyx—the equivalent of the deer's tail—will have to rotate in a smaller circle.

■ Make sure that you move from the waist and not from the shoulder.

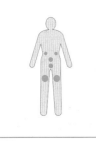

2 **Reach forward with your left hand, palm open and facing right. Keep your elbow slightly bent. Reach forward with your right hand, which should also be open and facing in, until it is parallel to your left elbow.**

RIGHT HAND IS PARALLEL TO THE LEFT ELBOW

● *The purpose of this exercise is to increase movement around your waist and tailbone (or coccyx) area, strengthening those regions and the kidneys, and improving circulation in the pelvic cavity. It also strengthens the legs.*

1

2

75%

75%

3 With your waist and the very end of your spine as the source of motion—not your shoulder joints—rotate your arms in a counterclockwise circle in front of your body. The circle drawn by your left hand will be greater than that drawn by your right hand. Repeat steps 1 to 3.

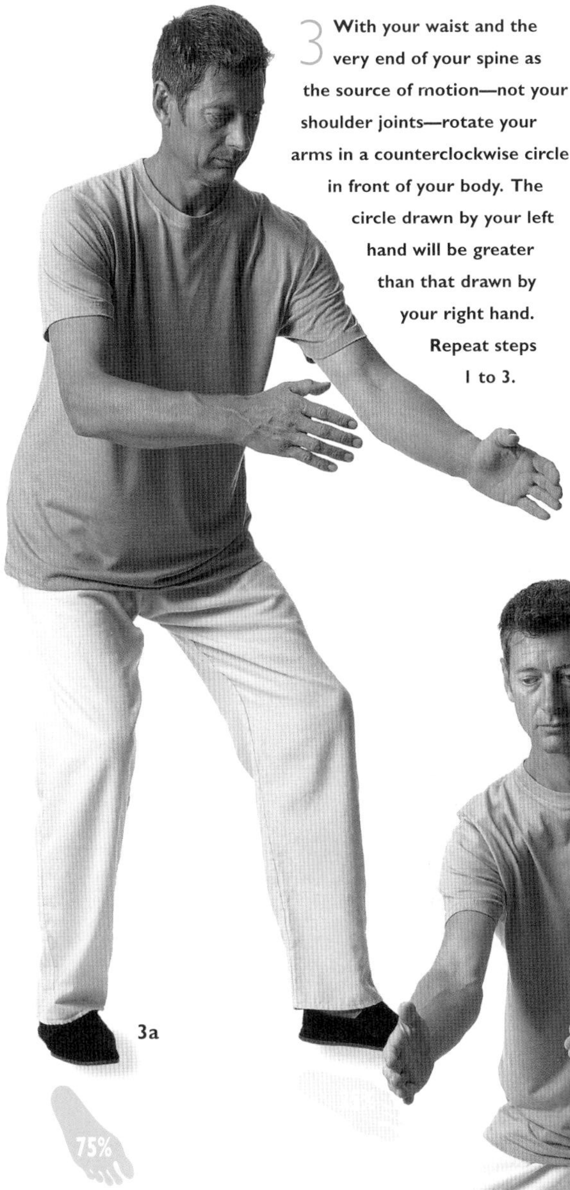

3a

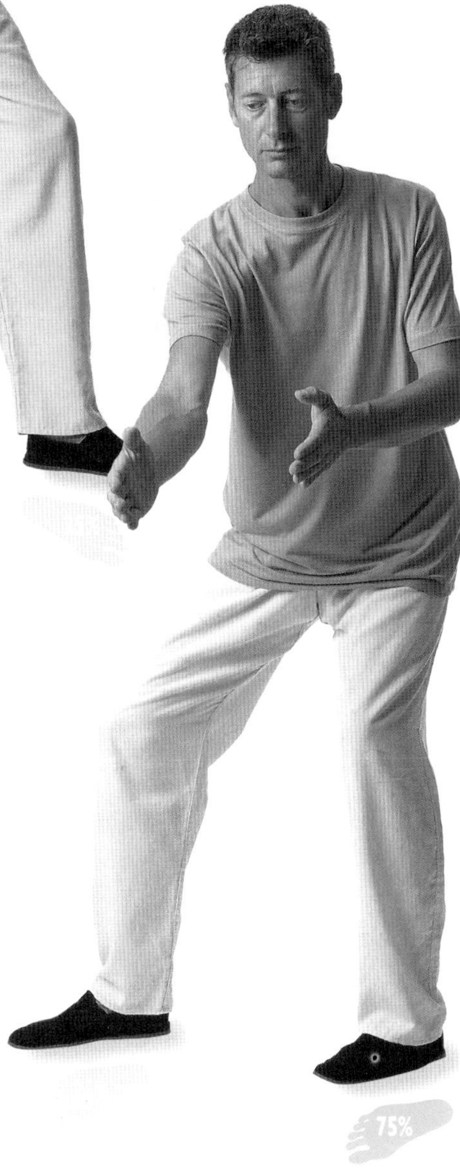

75%

3b

75%

REPEAT THE EXERCISE

4 Reverse the exercise. Step forward with your right foot while keeping your weight on your left. Reach your right hand forward with the palm open and your elbow slightly bent. Reach forward with your left hand in the same position until it is opposite your right elbow. Rotate your arms in a clockwise circle a number of times. Repeat the exercise in the opposite direction.

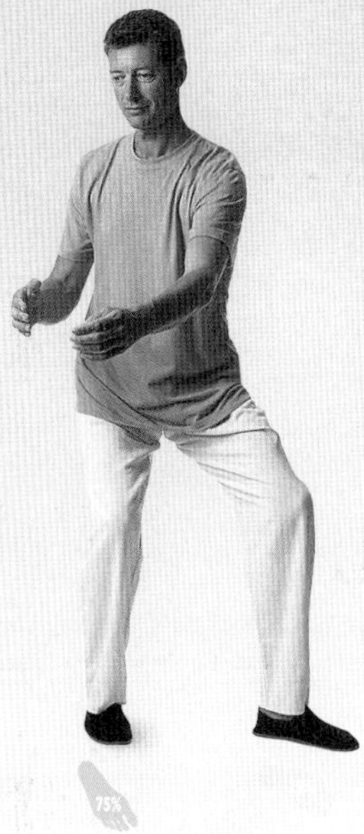

4a

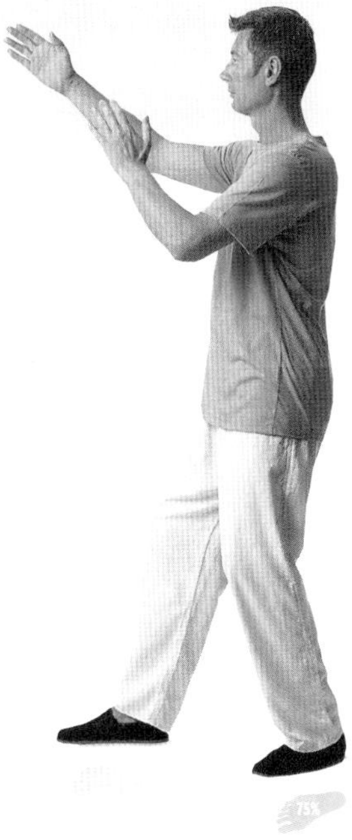

4b

SET 5 ▌ Bird play

Although it looks as though this exercise concerns the arms and legs, in reality it is the compression and expansion of the body that produces the beneficial effect of massaging and strengthening the heart, lungs, and kidneys.

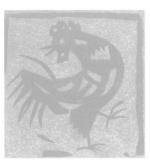

1 Stand with your arms hanging down naturally and your eyes looking straight ahead. Relax and remain calm for a few moments.

2 Step forward with your left foot. Follow with your right foot, but just take half a step. The toes of your right foot should gently touch the ground. As you take these steps, breathe in deeply and lift and spread your arms wide open in a large V.

3 Take a step forward with your right foot so that it lines up with your left foot. Then squat down and, as you do so, lower your arms, hug your knees and breathe out deeply.

ESSENTIAL POINTS

- Try to move gently and fluidly.
- Inhale as you stand up and open your arms.
- Exhale as you squat and hug your knees.

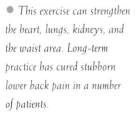

● *This exercise can strengthen the heart, lungs, kidneys, and the waist area. Long-term practice has cured stubborn lower back pain in a number of patients.*

1

2

3

4 As you stand up, take one step forward with your right foot and follow with a half step with your left foot. As you take these steps, sweep your arms open above your head in a large V and inhale.

REPEAT THE EXERCISE

5 Repeat steps 3 and 4, using opposite feet. Then repeat the whole sequence until you are pleasantly fatigued.

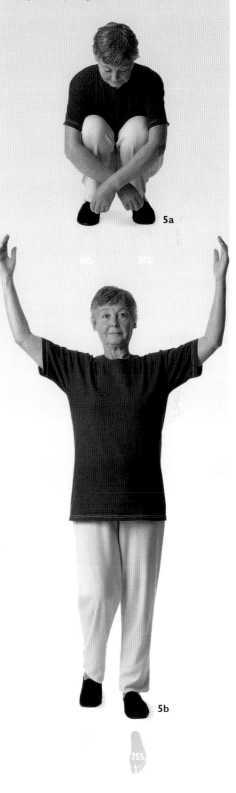

5a

5b

4

給每个人

2

YEE CHIN CHING

Strengthening with Yee Chin Ching

Yee Chin Ching was a popular fitness method in ancient China and although many centuries have passed, its popularity has not faded with time. Many people today practice Yee Chin Ching as part of their physical conditioning, and it is especially promoted by traditional Chinese doctors, who specialize in therapies based on postural alignment and massage and who do this exercise themselves.

Not only does Yee Chin Ching help promote good health and develop physical fitness and strength, but it can also be used as part of the recovery program for people suffering from bone-related ailments. It is especially effective in increasing muscular strength. Yee Chin Ching is thought to have been developed originally for training muscles and the tissues that line and connect them, the fascia. Literally *yee* means "transformation," *chin* means "muscles and tendons," and *ching*, "method." Yee Chin Ching is thus a method for transforming weak slack muscles and tendons into strong solid ones. The movements are similar to those of Pa Tuan Chin (*see pp. 48–55*), but Yee Chin is more demanding in terms of both strength and rigor of movement.

You need to maintain a tranquil mind, a composed mental spirit, and a harmonious breathing rhythm. In addition, you must attempt to unite motion with placidness and external force with internal force, or consciousness—*yi*.

One complete routine of Yee Chin Ching consists of 12 sets, which are described on the following pages. The movements of sets 1 to 3 follow each other and should be performed consecutively. Do each set only once.

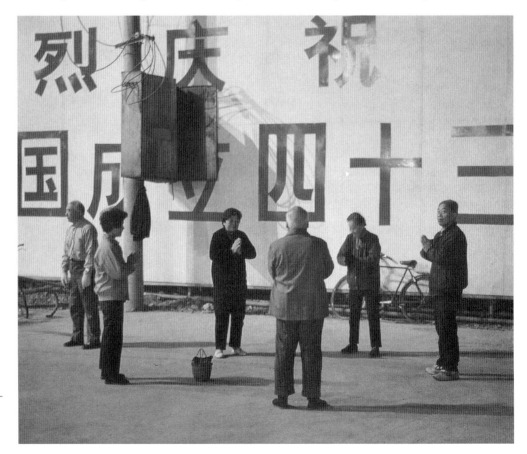

■ **Early-morning exercises being performed on the famous Bund in Shanghai.**

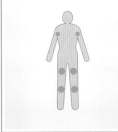

SET 1 | Folding hands in front of chest

Stand with your feet shoulder-width apart and your arms hanging naturally at your sides. Keep your back straight. Focus your eyes on distant objects and direct your full concentration on them. This is the starting position for all the forms that follow.

Leading with the backs of your open hands, raise your arms straight out in front of you, stopping at shoulder level. Your palms should be facing down.

1

2 **Turn your hands so that your palms face you,** with your finger tips almost touching. Draw your hands slowly toward you and stop about one fist away from your chest.

2

SET 2 | Raising arms to form a carrying pole

Begin in the standard relaxed, upright position, with your feet shoulder-width apart.

Grasp the ground with your toes. Turn your palms to face upward.

1

2 **As you rise on your toes, lift your arms straight out to the sides to shoulder level. Your palms should be up. Now sink back down on your feet, let your arms fall and relax.**

2

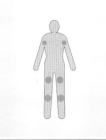

SET 3 | Holding the sky up with both hands

Assume the starting position, standing straight,
with your feet shoulder-width apart.

1 **Raise both arms slowly out to your sides with your palms facing up. Stretch them over your head, palms still up, and then turn them so your fingers are pointing inward and just touching as if you were holding up the sky. At the same time, lift your heels slightly off the ground, clench your teeth, touch your tongue to the roof of your mouth, and breathe deeply. Mentally concentrate on your hands.**

2 **Make your hands into fists and lower your arms from over your head to shoulder level out to the sides. At the same time, let your heels sink to the floor. You should move slowly, keeping muscular tension in your arms.**

ESSENTIAL POINTS

- Breathe deeply.
- Focus your attention on your hands, but don't actually look at them with your eyes.
- Maintain muscular tension in your arms.

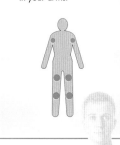

1

2

SET 4 | Exchanging one star for another

Continue from the previous form. Stand with your feet apart
and your arms out sidewise at shoulder level.

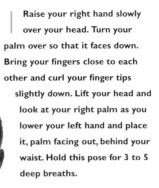

1 **Raise your right hand slowly
over your head. Turn your
palm over so that it faces down.
Bring your fingers close to each
other and curl your finger tips
slightly down. Lift your head and
look at your right palm as you
lower your left hand and place
it, palm facing out, behind your
waist. Hold this pose for 3 to 5
deep breaths.**

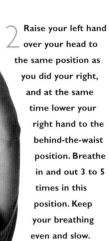

2 **Raise your left hand
over your head to
the same position as
you did your right,
and at the same
time lower your
right hand to the
behind-the-waist
position. Breathe
in and out 3 to 5
times in this
position. Keep
your breathing
even and slow.**

ESSENTIAL POINTS

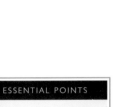

■ Look at your raised hand,
but concentrate on the
back of your waist where
your other hand is.

■ Breathe in and out
through your nose, or
breathe in through your
nose and out through
your mouth.

■ As you inhale, press your
waist gently with the back
of your hand. Release the
press as you exhale.

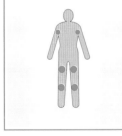

● *Do 3 to 5 complete repetitions
of this exercise.*

1

2

SET 5 ‖ Pulling the cow's tail backward

Continue from the pose that ended the previous form.

1 Withdraw your right hand from the rear of your waist and stretch it forward, turning it palm down. When your hand reaches shoulder level, bend your elbow slightly and bring your fingers together to form a "hook hand"—curl your fingers slightly in. Now take a long step forward with your right leg. Bend your right knee while keeping the left leg straight to form a sort of arch. At the same time, lower your left hand, form it into a loose fist, and draw it slightly behind your left hip. As you inhale, put your focus on your right hand and think of it as if it were pulling a cow's tail backward. As you exhale, put your attention on your left hand as though it were pushing the cow forward. Breathe in and out in this manner. Notice that your imaginary pulling backward and pushing forward are creating tension in your legs, trunk, shoulders, and elbows—they are meant to.

2 Swap the position of your left and right legs. With your left foot now in front and your knee bent, lift your left hand forward and form a hook hand. Bring your right hand just behind your right hip in a loose fist. Inhale and exhale, again pulling and pushing on the cow's tail.

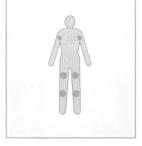

ESSENTIAL POINTS

- Keep your mental focus on each hand in turn, but look straight ahead.
- As you breathe, keep your lower abdomen comfortable and relaxed.
- The whole body should flex slightly.

● *Repeat the entire exercise 3 to 5 times.*

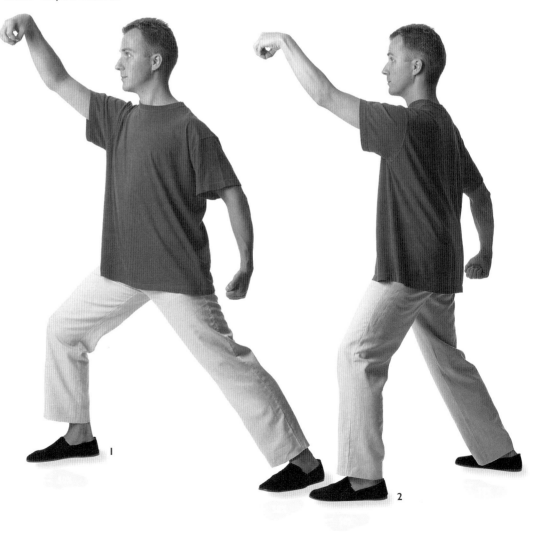

1

2

SET 6 | Pushing palms out to stretch arms

Start from the final position of the previous form. Bring your right foot forward to line up with your left foot, and stand up straight. Place both hands in front of your chest with your palms wide open and facing out and your fingers straight up.

1 Make "mountain-pushing" palms with your hands by keeping them at a 90-degree angle to your wrists, palms facing out. As you exhale, push out slowly from your chest with increasing force until your arms are fully extended. Keep your entire body straight, your eyes wide open, and your gaze on distant objects.

2 Slowly return your hands to the position in front of your chest, inhaling as you do so.

ESSENTIAL POINTS

■ Exert force gradually.

■ When your palms reach their full extension, the force is almost powerful enough to push down an imaginary mountain— hence the name of the hand position.

■ Keep your breathing rhythm harmonious— exhale while pushing forward, inhale while bringing the hands back.

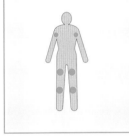

● *Repeat the entire exercise 3 to 5 times.*

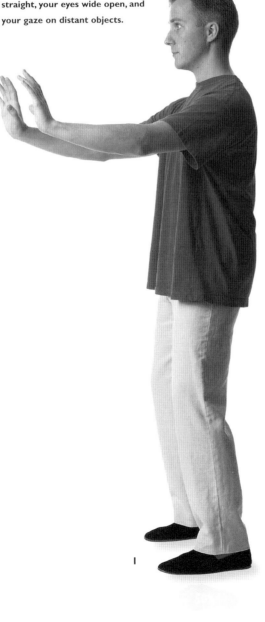

1

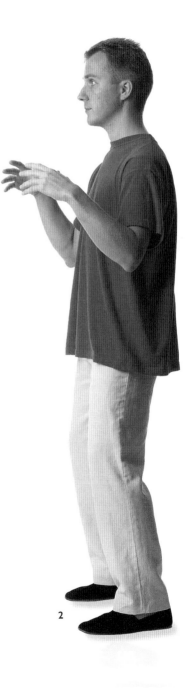

2

SET 7 ▌ Drawing a sword

Start from the previous form with your arms extended at shoulder
level and your palms in the mountain-pushing position.

1 | Clasp the back of your head with your right hand.
**Pull on your left ear gently, but keep your elbow
back. Turn your head to the left, lower your left hand,
and, with your palm out, bring it up between your
shoulder blades as far as you can. As you breathe in,
tug and squeeze your left ear with your right hand,
keeping your elbow back and your neck straight.
Concentrate on your right elbow. Breathe out and
relax the pressure on your ear. Breathe in and out in
this position 3 to 5 times.**

2 | **Raise your right hand up and put it between your
shoulder blades, palm facing out. At the same
time, put the palm of your left hand at the back of
your head. Pull your right ear gently with your fingers.
Keep your elbow back and your head turned to the
right. As you breathe in, squeeze and pull on your
right ear with your hand. Keep your left elbow pulled
back and your attention focused on it. Relax and
exhale. Breathe in and out and repeat your ear pulling
and elbow stretching 3 to 5 times.**

ESSENTIAL POINTS

■ Keep your body
straight—do not allow
your back to twist.

■ Breathe freely throughout
the exercise.

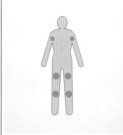

● *Repeat the entire exercise on
both sides 3 to 5 times.*

1

2

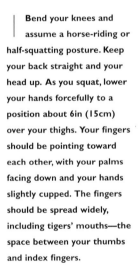

SET 8 ‖ Planting feet solidly on the ground

Stand in a relaxed at-attention pose. Take a large step to the left so that your feet are wider apart than your shoulders. Raise your arms out to the sides, to shoulder level, palms down.

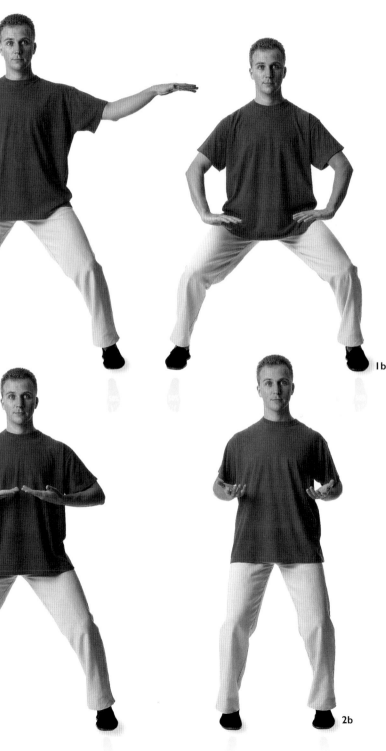

1 Bend your knees and assume a horse-riding or half-squatting posture. Keep your back straight and your head up. As you squat, lower your hands forcefully to a position about 6in (15cm) over your thighs. Your fingers should be pointing toward each other, with your palms facing down and your hands slightly cupped. The fingers should be spread widely, including tigers' mouths—the space between your thumbs and index fingers.

2 Turn your palms over and slowly but forcefully raise them to chest level as if you were lifting a 1000lb (450kg) weight. Then rise up from your squat at the same slow pace, and turn your fingers to face away from you.

● *Repeat the entire exercise 3 to 5 times.*

1a

1b

2a

2b

SET 9 | Throwing fists from left and right

Stand in the usual starting position, a relaxed at-attention posture with your feet shoulder-width apart and your back straight. Bend your elbows back slightly and open your hands with palms up.

1 **Turn your hands over and make loose fists. Bend your** elbows slightly and bring your fists up to the sides of your waist. Then slowly swing your right fist out toward the left, letting your upper body turn with the motion. Simultaneously draw your left elbow back and turn the fist up.

2 **When you reach the end of the swing, reverse directions.** Start withdrawing your right fist back to your side, ending with the fist up, as you begin to swing your left fist out to the right, ending with the fist down, as in step 1.

ESSENTIAL POINTS

■ The fist throwing and withdrawing should all be part of one smooth continuous sweep. The withdrawing and extending motions are like waves, steady and uninterrupted.

■ Your breathing should also be coordinated. Breathe in through your nose while swinging your fist out and exhale when it is fully extended.

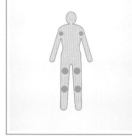

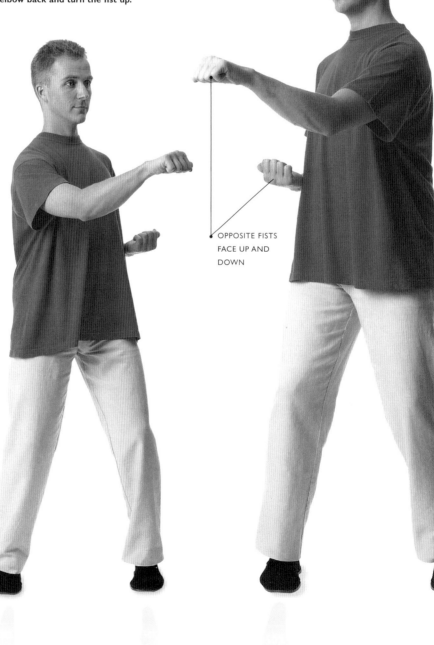

OPPOSITE FISTS FACE UP AND DOWN

● *Repeat this 3 to 5 times.* 1

2

SET 10 ┃ Catching prey like a fierce tiger

Stand in a relaxed at-attention pose and let your arms hang down naturally.

1 Take a large step forward with your right foot, bend your right knee, and extend your left leg far behind you. At the same time, lean forward onto your fingers. You will now be in a position similar to a sprinter about to start a race. Keep your head up and your gaze fixed straight ahead.

2 Bend your arms at the elbows and move your body slightly forward. Move slowly. Imagine that you are a fierce tiger stalking its prey. Then raise your upper body, straightening your elbows, and simultaneously move slightly backward. Repeat this whole sequence 3 to 5 times. Stand up and bring your right foot back to its original position.

3 Now take one large step forward with your left foot and repeat steps 1 and 2.

4 Return to your starting posture. Do this exercise only once with each leg.

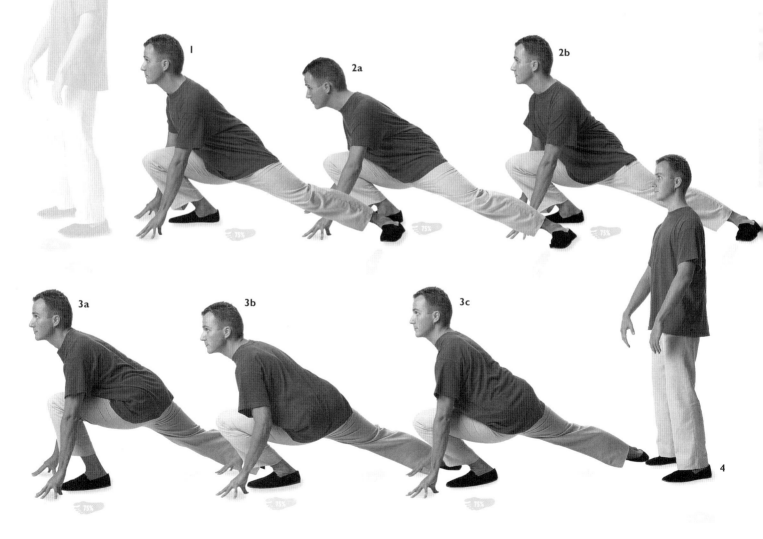

SET 11 | Bowing the body

Stand in a relaxed at-attention pose and let your arms hang down naturally.

1 **Wrap your fingers around the back of your head and lace your fingers together. Stretch your elbows to the rear.**

2 **Bow forward from the waist, keeping your knees straight. Your head is lowered as if you were giving a bow. Keep your knees straight.**

3 **In this position, do the exercise called beating heaven's drum. Unlace your hands and place the bottom of your palms over your ears. Place each index finger on top of the middle finger of the same** hand, then let the index fingers slide off to strike your head. Drum 10 to 20 times. Your fingers are hitting below the occipital cavity on either side of the spine, also known as the Feng Chih acupuncture point. According to traditional Chinese medicine, this point is part of the Foot-Lesser Yang-Gall Bladder Meridian. Applying acupuncture techniques to this point can treat headache, dizziness, and stiffness of the neck and collarbone area. Striking the Feng Chih point with the index finger is in essence massaging this point with the point-rapping technique.

ESSENTIAL POINTS

■ Do not bend more than you comfortably can.

■ Keep your teeth loosely clenched and your tongue gently touching the roof of your mouth.

■ Breathe lightly or hold your breath until you straighten up again.

● *In the beginning, repeat the bow only once or twice. Later, you may gradually increase this to 3 to 5 times.*

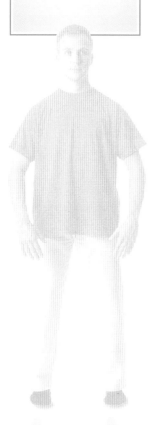

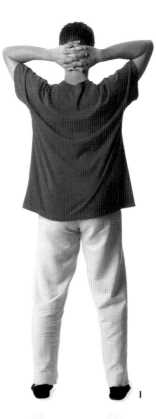

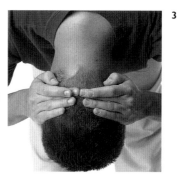

3

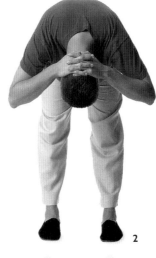

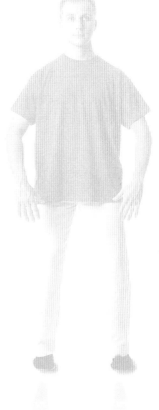

1

2

SET 12 | Wagging the tail

Stand in the starting position, loosely at attention with your arms
hanging naturally.

1 **Raise your hands to the front
of your chest and push out**
with slightly cupped palms until
your arms are fully extended.

2 **Bring your hands back to your
chest and interlock your**
fingers, with the palms facing down.

3 **Lean forward and try to touch
the floor with your palms.**
Do not force your body to bend,
however. Lift your head slightly.
Keep your eyes wide open and fix
your gaze straight ahead.

4 **Straighten up, unlace your
fingers and reach for the sky,**
rising up on your toes as you do
so. As you sink down onto your
soles again, lower your arms down
to your sides.

ESSENTIAL POINTS

■ Breathe naturally, exhaling
as you bend forward and
inhaling as you straighten
up again.

■ Bend as far as you
comfortably can. Don't
worry if you can't reach
the floor at first; this will
become easier, the more
you practice

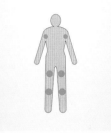

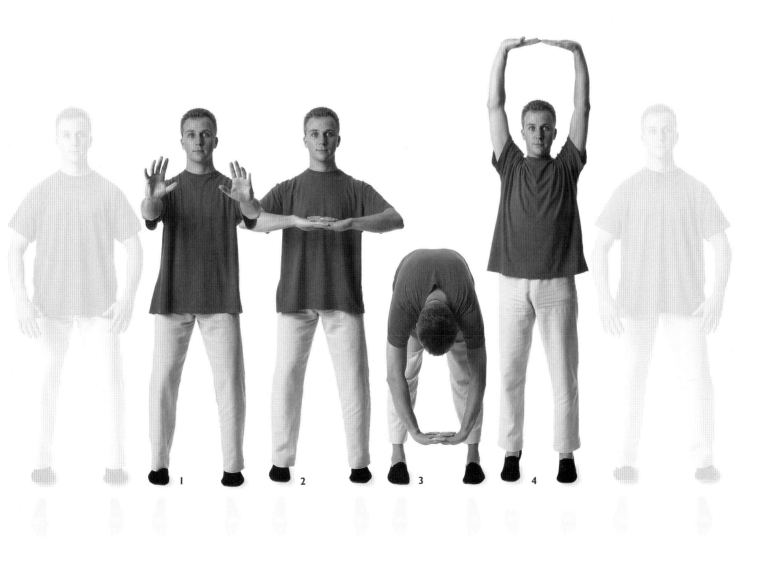

給每个人

（3）

PA TUAN CHIN

The Eight Sets of Embroidery

Chin is an embroidered work of silks in various colors. The ancient Chinese, more than 800 years ago, broadened the meaning of *chin* to include certain carefully selected and compiled sets of exercises. Pa Tuan Chin consists of eight sets of movements.

Pa Tuan Chin can be performed in either the standing or the bent-knee, horse-riding position. Although it involves moving the trunk, head, and neck, its main emphasis is on the arms. It can help increase arm and leg strength, develop the chest, and prevent incorrect posture such as saddleback or a rounded back, in young and old alike. There are two approaches—movement with force and movement without force. When it is performed with force, the force should be steady, even, and potential, rather than overt.

There is no limit to the number of repetitions of each set. You may do 8 to 16 or as many as you like. But once you have decided, do the same number of repetitions for all the sets of Pa Tuan Chin. Continuous smooth movement of the body will encourage the *chi* to flow.

SET 1 ▌ Holding up the sky with both hands

Stand to attention with your arms hanging naturally. Look straight ahead.

1 **Slowly raise your arms out to the sides, then over your head.** With your palms down, lace your fingers together as you lift your heels about 1in (2.5cm) off the ground.

2 **Turn your palms over, keeping your elbows straight. Press up with your hands as you lift your heels farther off the ground. Now** hold this pose for a few seconds.

3 **Release your fingers and slowly bring your arms down** sidewise, but keep your heels off the ground.

4 **Bring your heels down gently to the ground and return to** the starting position.

ESSENTIAL POINTS

- Look straight ahead throughout.
- Keep your breathing steady, exhaling as you press up and inhaling as you bring your arms down again.

1   2   3   4

SET 2 | Drawing a bow

Stand in a relaxed at-attention posture.

1 Take one step to the left and bend your legs to assume a horse-riding posture. Your thighs should be as close to being parallel to the ground as possible. Your back should be straight. Cross your arms in front of your chest with your right arm out and left arm in. Your fingers should be loosely separated. Turn your head to the left and look at your right hand.

2 Make a fist with your left hand. Extend both your index finger and your thumb while keeping the other three fingers curled. Slowly uncurl your left arm to the left until it is fully extended and, at the same time, make your right hand into a fist and draw it to the right, as if you were pulling a bow. Your right elbow should be pointing right. Your eyes should be focused on your left index finger.

3 Relax your left hand and bring it back to the front of your chest at the same time as you are bringing your right hand back. Cross both arms again, this time with your left arm out and your right arm in. Turn to the right and look at your left hand.

4 Make a fist with your right hand. Extend your index finger and thumb while keeping the other three fingers curled. Slowly uncurl your right arm to the right until it is fully extended; at the same time make a fist with your left hand and draw the elbow to the left as though pulling a bow. Your eyes should stay on your right index finger.

ESSENTIAL POINTS

■ Try to keep your thighs parallel to the ground, but keep your feet flat on the floor.

■ Don't forget to change your focus from your folded hand to the extended index finger on the opposite hand.

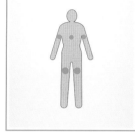

SET 3 | Lifting a single hand

Stand loosely to attention with your arms hanging naturally at your sides and your feet flat on the ground and positioned so that they are close together. Look straight ahead of you.

1 **Flex your left hand back toward the wrist, keeping your fingers together and your elbow straight. Raise the arm out to the left and then over your head. Your palm should be up and your fingers pointing right. At the same time, stretch your right hand down toward the floor, with your palm facing back.**

2 **Bring your left hand down in a slow semicircle to the left, and stretch it toward the floor with your palm facing back. At the same time, flex your right hand back toward your wrist and raise it in a slow semicircle to the right until it is over your head. Your palm is now facing up, your fingers are together and pointing left, and your arm is fully extended.**

ARM IS EXTENDED
UNTIL IT IS STRAIGHT

OPPOSITE ARM IS THEN
RAISED AND EXTENDED

ESSENTIAL POINTS

■ Extend both arms until they are straight.
■ Move slowly.
■ Take care not to twist your torso.

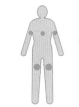

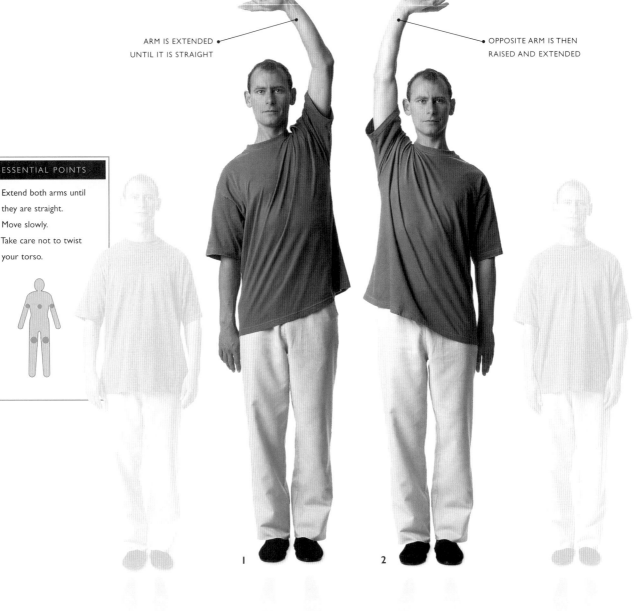

1

2

SET 4 | Looking backward

Stand in a relaxed at-attention posture. Hold your head up straight. Let your
arms hang naturally, but press your palms tightly against your outer thighs.

1 **Keep your chest upright and
pull your shoulders slightly
back. At the same time, turn your
head slowly to the left and look
behind you.**

2 **Relax your head and shoulders,
then turn to the front again,
and look straight ahead of you.**

3 **Keep your chest upright and
pull your shoulders slightly
back. At the same time, turn your
head slowly to the right and look
behind you.**

4 **Bring your head and shoulders
back to the starting position
and look straight ahead.**

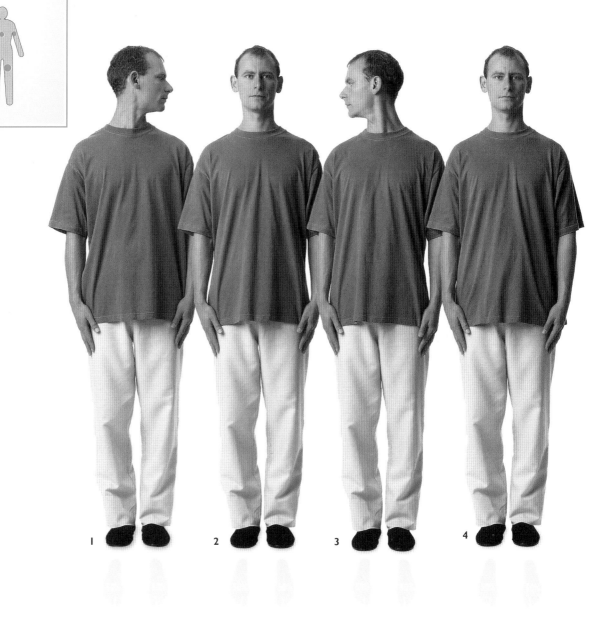

1   2   3   4

SET 5 | Wagging head and tail

Stand with your feet wide apart, at a distance equal to about three times the length of one of your feet. Bend your knees and assume a horse-riding posture. Place your hands just above your knees with your tigers' mouths—the space between your thumbs and index fingers—facing in toward your body. Keep your upper body straight.

1 Bend your upper body low to the left front with your head down. Swing your head and upper body in a clockwise circle in front of you. You will find that as your head circles, so do your buttocks. This is head and tail wagging.

2 Stop the circle when you are leaning right, and return to the starting position—squatting as if riding a horse but with your back straight.

3 Bend your upper body low to the left front and circle counterclockwise. Stop circling, but remain in the horse-riding posture for a moment or two.

ESSENTIAL POINTS

■ As you circle, your weight transfers from one leg to the other.

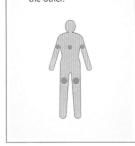

1

2a

2b

3

SET 6 | Touching toes with both hands

Stand in a relaxed at-attention posture.

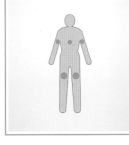

1 | Bend your upper body slowly forward with your knees straight and touch your toes or ankles. Keep your head very slightly raised.

2 Straighten up and return to the starting position.

3 Place your hands in the small of your back. Slowly and carefully bend backward.

4 Straighten up and return to the starting position.

BACK-BEND IS SUPPORTED BY THE HANDS ●

BODY BENDS FORWARD FROM THE HIPS ●

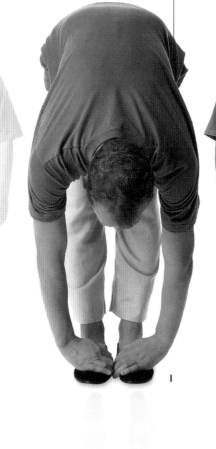

1

2

3

4

SET 7 ▮ Holding fists and opening angry eyes

Stand with your feet more than shoulder-width apart. Bend your knees and assume a horse-riding posture. Place your fists at the sides of your waist, fingers facing up.

1 **Extend your left arm slowly forward until your fist is straight out in front of you, fingers facing down. At the same time, clench your right fist tightly and pull your elbow to the rear. Open your eyes wide and glare at objects in front of you for a moment.**

2 **Draw both fists back to the sides of your waist, with your fingers facing up again. Repeat the exercise, reversing the position of your arms.**

3 **Return to the starting position with both of your fists at your sides.**

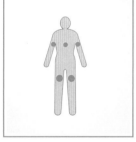

ESSENTIAL POINTS

■ Try not to blink as you stare at objects in front of you.

■ Relax your eyes when you return both your fists to your sides.

■ Do the exercise in one smooth, continuous motion, but remember to move slowly.

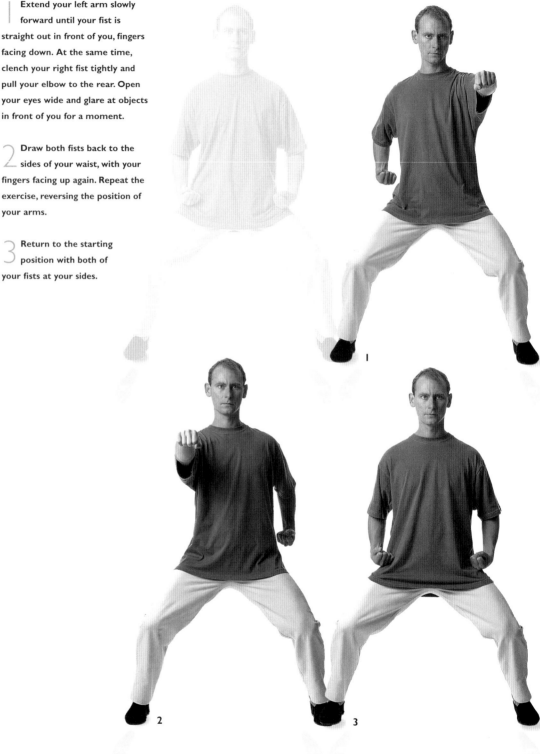

1

2

3

SET 8 ▌ Jolting the back

Stand to attention, with your feet together and your palms flat against your thighs.

1 **Stand up very straight. Propel your head straight up by lifting your heels high off the ground.**

2 **Lower your heels quite quickly and stand in the starting position again.**

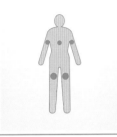

ESSENTIAL POINTS

■ Keep your head straight when you are standing on tiptoe—don't let it tilt forward.

■ Lower your heels suddenly to get the "jolt" in your back.

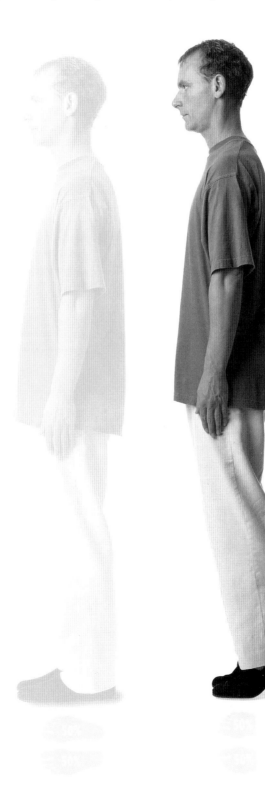

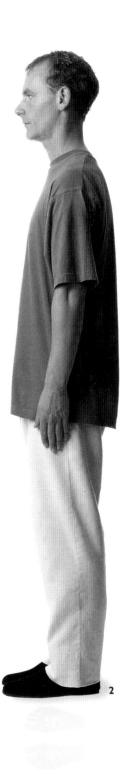

1

2

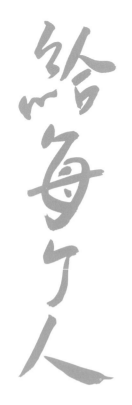

(4)

SHIH ERH TUAN CHIN

The Twelve Sets of Embroidery

A remarkably effective exercise, Shih Erh Tuan Chin has been practiced in China for many centuries. It consists of self-massage and fitness exercises, which can also be done by the old and weak or those suffering from chronic diseases. The first 11 sets can be performed in a cross-legged position or seated; the last set in a standing position.

SET 1 | Teeth tapping

Tap your upper and lower teeth against each other 20 to 30 times. This helps stimulate the blood vessels in your gums, improving circulation in the area and strengthening your teeth. It also helps prevent dental disease.

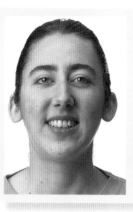

SET 2 | Tongue revolving

Move the tip of your tongue against your teeth in all directions—left and right, up and down, front and back. Do this until your mouth feels tingly. This exercise has a massaging effect on the gums and the mucous membrane of the mouth cavity, contributing to successful treatment of bleeding and receding gums. It also keeps the mouth cavity clean, stimulates the secretion of saliva, and speeds up digestion. Try not to swallow until you have done the exercise, then relax your stomach while swallowing the accumulated saliva. This will aid the functioning of the gastro-intestinal tract.

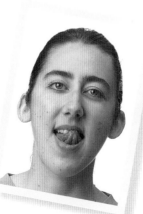

SET 3 | Face rubbing

First rub your palms rapidly together to create some warmth and bring *chi* to them. Then lightly rub your face with your palms 20 to 30 times as follows: from the nose across the cheeks to the ears; from the bridge of the nose across the forehead to the ears; and from the chin up the jaws to the ears. This action can help improve blood circulation in the skin and help maintain elasticity.

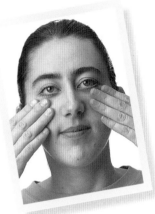

SET 4 | Beating heaven's drum

Cover your ears with the base of your palms and place your index fingers on top of your middle fingers. Then let your index fingers slide off so that they strike the back of your head in the vicinity of the Feng Chih (Windy Lake) acupuncture point (Gall Bladder 20, *see also p. 46, step 3*). Do this 20 to 30 times. You will hear a drumlike sound.

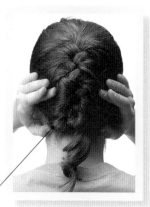

GALL BLADDER 20
ACUPUNCTURE POINT

SET 5 ▌ Wheel-turning

Make your hands into fists over your head with your knuckles pointing forward. Bend your elbows slightly and bring your arms forward and back as if you were spinning a water wheel. Do this 10 or more times. This exercise is effective in preventing arthritic changes in the shoulder joints.

SET 6 ▌ Holding up the sky

Clasp your hands with your fingers interlocked in front of you. Turn your palms over and stretch your arms above your head as if you were holding up the sky. Do this 10 or more times. This exercise can help to expand your chest and facilitate deep breathing.

SET 7 ▌ Drawing a bow in two directions

Mimic the motions of drawing and shooting a bow (see p. 49, steps 2, 3, and 4 – arm movements only). In order to activate the relevant meridians, try to get your index finger to point straight up. Alternate both hands and sides. Do this 10 or more times. This exercise stretches and expands your chest, as well as training your shoulder joints and adding strength to your arms.

SET 8 | Lowering the head and touching the toes

Sit on the floor with your legs fully extended. Lean forward and touch your toes with your hands. Do this 10 or more times. Since this exercise involves moving the waist and abdomen, it is relatively demanding. It stretches the muscles in your waist, back, and thighs, as well as contributing to flexibility in the spine and to the overall health of your body.

YUNG CHUAN, OR KIDNEY 1, IS LOCATED ONE-THIRD OF THE WAY DOWN THE FOOT

SET 9 | Rubbing Tan Tien (Field of the Elixir)

Tan Tien is generally believed to be located about 3in (7.5cm) below the navel. Rubbing Tan Tien is in essence rubbing your lower abdomen and you will probably also be rubbing the Shih Men (Stone Gate) point which, according to Chinese medicine, is part of Jen Mo (The Conception Vessel), an acupuncture meridian. Rub the lower abdomen in a circular motion with three fingers of your right hand for 30 or more rotations. Choose the direction according to which of the following options sounds most appropriate for you. Rubbing in a clockwise direction (as you look at your abdomen) will strengthen the genitourinary section, reducing involuntary seminal emissions caused by weak intestinal energy. It will also invigorate the circulation of blood and *chi* in the lower body cavity, promoting strength in the internal organs. Counterclockwise rubbing will reduce abdominal pain, discomfort, and indigestion.

TAN TIEN IS FOUND JUST BELOW THE NAVEL

SET 10 ▮ Rubbing Shen Yu (Respectable Kidney)

Rub your hands briskly together to create warmth and bring *chi* to the palms. Then place your palms against the back of your waist, over the kidneys, to massage the Shen Yu points located here. Rub at least 20 to 30 times. While massaging these points, imagine warm energy leaving the center of your palms and entering the kidneys. This exercise is helpful in preventing lower back pain and improving your health in general.

HANDS MASSAGE THE
SHEN YU POINT IN THE
SMALL OF THE BACK

SET 12 ▮ Foot treading

You do this exercise standing up. Plant one foot at a time firmly on the ground, one after the other. Inhale as you lift your foot and exhale as you plant it on the ground. Do this 10 or more times. This exercise can revitalize blood circulation as well as stretch the muscles and supportive tissues of the leg.

FEET ARE LIFTED AND
LOWERED ALTERNATELY

SET 11 ▮ Rubbing Yung Chuan (Bubbling Spring)

First rub your hands together to create warmth and bring *chi* to the palms. Then rub the sole of your left foot with the three middle fingers of your right hand until heat is generated. Next rub the sole of your right foot with your left hand in the same way. According to traditional Chinese medicine, Yung Chuan, which is located one-third of the way down the foot, in the depression formed when the toes are curled under (Kidney 1), is the starting point of the Foot-Lesser Yin-Kidney Meridian. Massaging this point can cause so-called deficiency heat to descend. This assists in the treatment of insomnia, menopausal hot flushes, and heart palpitations. It can also improve your walking.

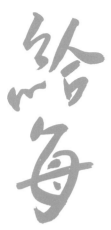

An Introduction to Tai Chi Chuan

Tai Chi Chuan (Yin-Yang Boxing) is believed to have been created by the Taoist monk Chang San Feng about 800 years ago. It was originally a form of martial art, used for self-defense purposes, but is now most widely known as a self-healing and self-development system. It is a form of Chi Kung (self-healing or energy exercises) from which everyone can benefit.

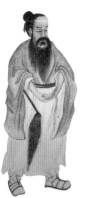

■ **Chang San Feng reputedly developed Tai Chi after a dream involving a fight between a bird and a snake.**

■ **Tai Chi is characterized by gentle, flowing movements that anyone can perform.**

Centuries of successful use of Tai Chi Chuan, often abbreviated to Tai Chi, testify to the health-improving benefits of this gentle flowing system, also known as Yin-Yang Boxing. To know Tai Chi fully, you should study with someone who has already mastered the art. It involves memorizing, over a period of time, a graceful dancelike routine, which will result in the progressive learning of the proper attitude of relaxation. But if there are no Tai Chi classes near you or if you prefer to work alone, you can still get most of the benefits of this splendid exercise.

Tai Chi involves the whole body. It can help everyone—male or female, old or young, fit or weak—develop grace, coordination, and balance. Each movement strengthens and tones a different group of muscles, tendons, and joints. Consistent practice makes joints more flexible and ligaments more elastic. It also increases muscular strength. Most importantly, Tai Chi increases the amount of *chi* energy in the body and improves its circulation through the acupuncture meridian system, leading to good health and longevity.

Tai Chi breathing must be deep but quiet, long but rhythmic. Because the breathing and movements stimulate the waist region in particular, blood circulation in the abdomen is enhanced, and stomach and intestinal movement are speeded up.

EXERCISE FROM TAI CHI

People who have not successfully learned the whole Tai Chi routine may practice Tai Chi movement exercises instead. In essence, this is a freestyle exercise that you invent as you go along,

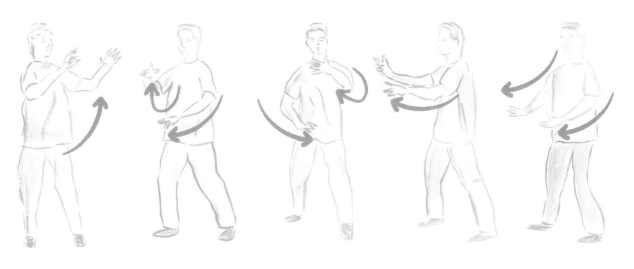

and which is based loosely on the grace, fluidity, slowness, and softness of Tai Chi. However, it is much easier to learn and do, so it has a greater appeal for some people.

You need to relax your entire body, including the respiratory muscles, and breathe naturally. The speed and frequency of your breathing should be allowed to follow their natural course. Breathe in and out through your nose, or in through your nose and out through your mouth. Concentrate mentally. To reduce distractions, you may leave your eyes partially closed or fully open, whichever is most relaxing for you. Gently focus your attention on the area of your navel.

Once your body is completely relaxed, you can start to make gentle movements. Keep your knees slightly bent whenever your body is in motion. You may move your body any way you want, in approximate imitation of the movements of Tai Chi (*see pp.* 62–67). Let your trunk, arms, and legs move freely, without the slightest restraint. After practicing for a period of time, the movement will become increasingly spontaneous. Do not be concerned about performing any special movements or deliberately seeking them. Let them come naturally.

When you want to end the exercise, do so slowly. After stopping, walk for a few minutes and breathe deeply a few times. Alternatively, massage your head for a while.

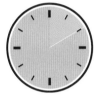

■ The whole Tai Chi set may take up to 10 minutes.

THE NAVEL BECOMES THE MAIN POINT OF FOCUS

KNEES ARE FLEXED SLIGHTLY TO ASSIST MOVEMENT

■ A straight and vertical spine is one of the most essential elements of Tai Chi Chuan.

ESSENTIALS OF TAI CHI

◆ A whole set of simplified Tai Chi (*see pp. 62–67*) usually takes 4 to 6 minutes, but it is fine to take as long as 8 or 9 minutes and do it in slow motion.

◆ To get the best results, you need a vision of how the exercise should be practiced. See yourself moving your body softly and breathing in and out naturally. The movements must be continuous, soft, slow, gentle, measured, and smooth. You must try to walk like a cat and move like silk off the reel.

◆ Beginners should breathe naturally. Do not breathe hard, pant, or hold breath.

◆ After you have become proficient, you may coordinate movements with your breathing. Exhale as your hands move away from your body; inhale as your hands move toward you. Breathe with your abdomen, deeply and naturally.

◆ Relax your entire body and keep your posture natural and comfortable. It is especially important to relax the waist, abdomen, and chest muscles. Maintain a good balance between activity and placidness. Artificial force should not be applied.

◆ Let your back muscles stretch out and your shoulders hang naturally. Let your elbows relax. This posture will enable you to feel natural and to maintain a stable center of gravity.

◆ Concentrate fully on the movements and avoid distractions. You need to be mentally quiet and peaceful.

◆ The goal is to integrate *hsing* (physical form) with *yi* (concentration) and to guide your body movements with your mind, visualizing the form as you do it.

◆ Force and power must be internally restrained and not externally revealed. The muscles should never be tensed to create force and power.

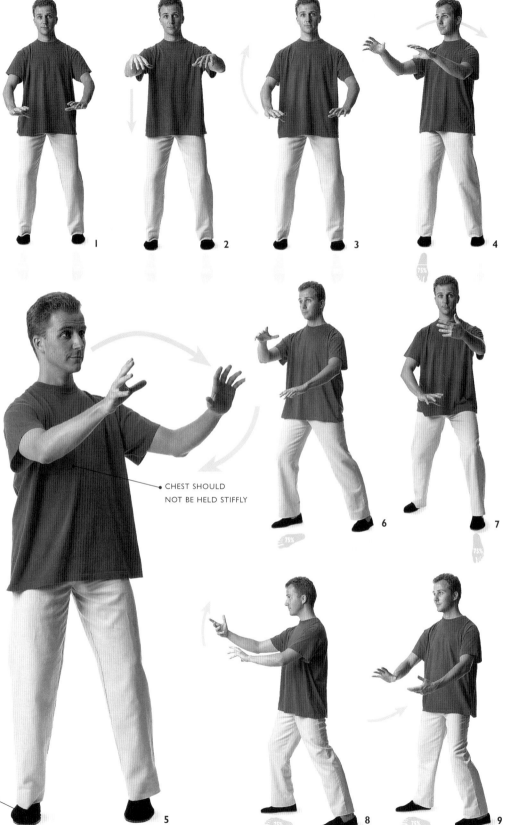

Steps 1 to 15 involve movements mainly of the arms and hands, while the position of the feet and distribution of the body's weight shift only slightly.

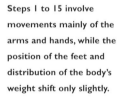

CHEST SHOULD NOT BE HELD STIFFLY

FEET ARE PARALLEL AND SHOULDER-WIDTH APART

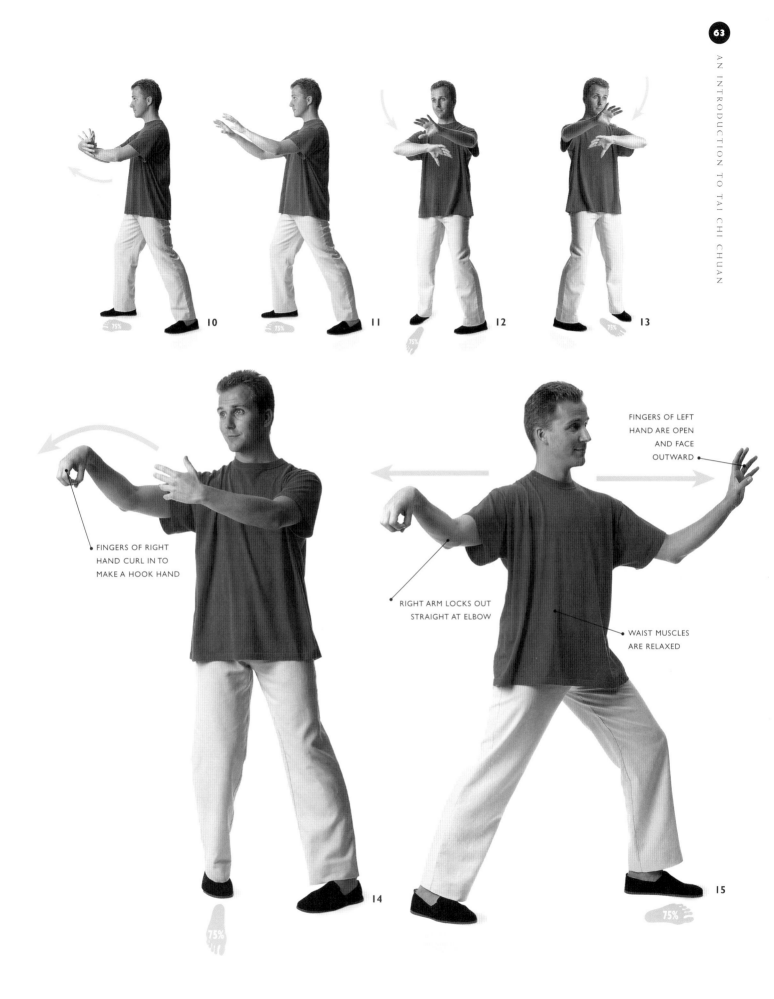

10

11

12

13

FINGERS OF RIGHT
HAND CURL IN TO
MAKE A HOOK HAND

14

FINGERS OF LEFT
HAND ARE OPEN
AND FACE
OUTWARD

RIGHT ARM LOCKS OUT
STRAIGHT AT ELBOW

WAIST MUSCLES
ARE RELAXED

15

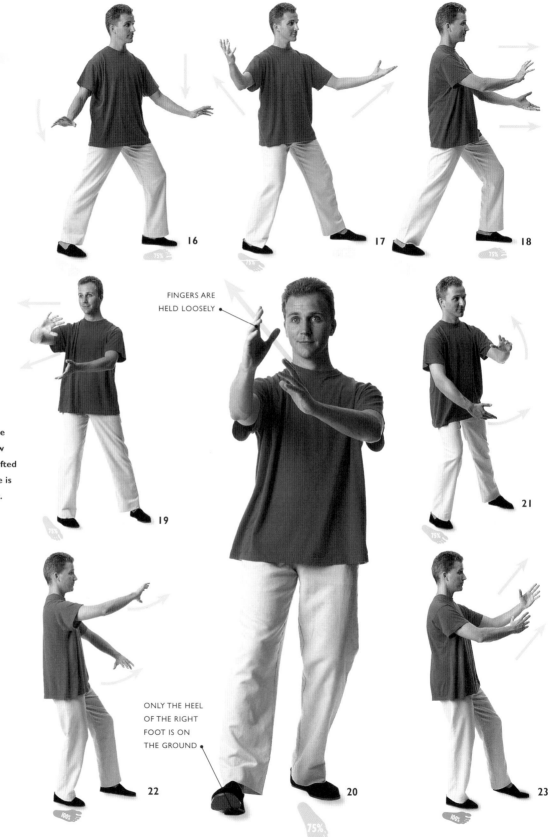

16

17

18

FINGERS ARE
HELD LOOSELY •

Steps 16 to 32 involve
further movement of the
arms and hands, but now
one foot is sometimes lifted
from the floor and there is
a greater shift of weight.

19

21

ONLY THE HEEL
OF THE RIGHT
FOOT IS ON
THE GROUND •

22

20

23

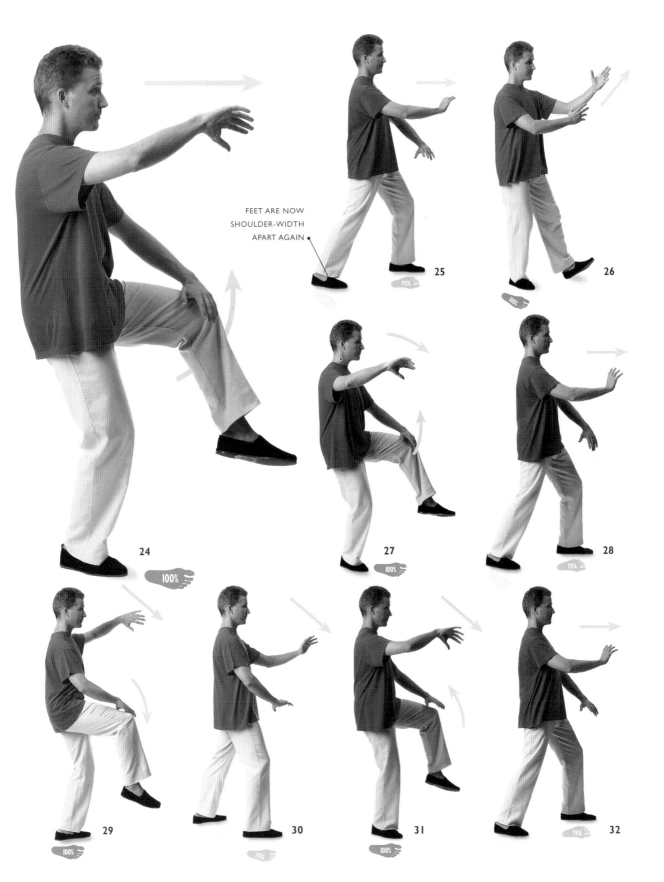

FEET ARE NOW
SHOULDER-WIDTH
APART AGAIN

24 100%

25 75%

26 100%

27 100%

28 75%

29 100%

30 75%

31 100%

32 75%

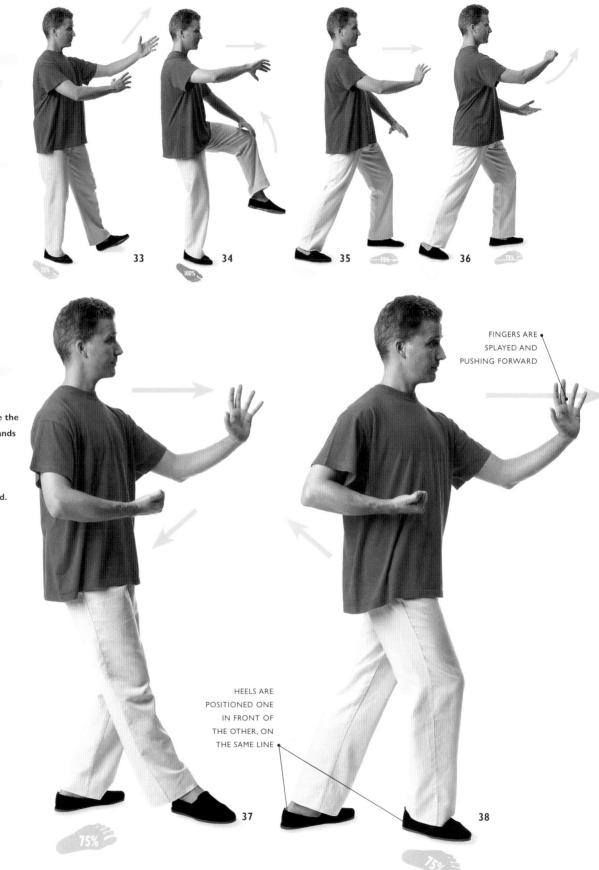

33

34

35

36

Steps 33 to 46 involve the movement of both hands and feet, finishing in exactly the same position in which the exercises were started.

FINGERS ARE SPLAYED AND PUSHING FORWARD

HEELS ARE POSITIONED ONE IN FRONT OF THE OTHER, ON THE SAME LINE

37

38

75%

75%

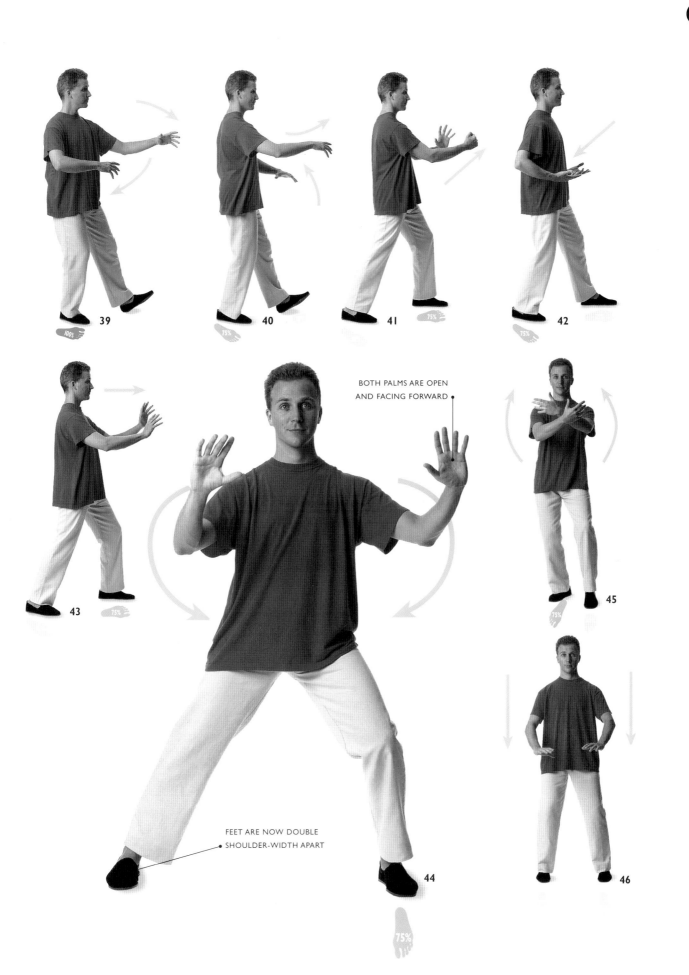

39

40

41

42

43

BOTH PALMS ARE OPEN
AND FACING FORWARD

45

FEET ARE NOW DOUBLE
SHOULDER-WIDTH APART

44

46

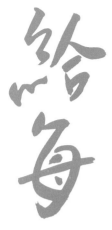

An Introduction to Chi Kung

Chi Kung means literally "energy exercises." To be healthy our chi, or life force, must be full, flowing and balanced, for a deficiency of chi will lead to a lowered body resistance to disease; stagnated chi will lead to obstruction and impaired function of the body's organs; and an imbalance of chi will lead to irregularities of the body's internal systems.

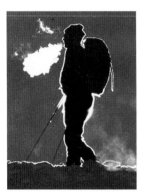

■ **Conquering any physical or mental task can be termed a form of kung fu.**

Chi Kung is a kung fu—mastery of a mental or physical feat through systematic practice. It is designed to train or condition *chi*, or energy. In Chinese medicine, *chi* refers both to the air you inhale and to yuen chi—the primary vital energy stored in the body. To condition *chi* is, in essence, to condition yuen chi. Yuen chi may be considered to be roughly equivalent to the sum total of the body's ability to resist disease, to adapt to the external environment, and to restore proper internal functioning. Chi Kung both conditions and nourishes this vital energy to improve physical stamina and health.

In general, Chi Kung consists of three interdependent parts, relating to the body, mind, and breathing, which you need to develop together in order to learn the basic techniques.

Chi Kung adjusts your body posture. You must be relaxed and natural. To relax your body, loosen your belt and clothes. Make sure that your shoulders are not raised or your chest elevated. You should not try too hard to hold your body in an unnatural pose. If you don't feel comfortable with a posture, you should adjust yourself so that you are free from any constraints. Above all, you must relax your muscles, particularly those of the lower abdomen, so that the *chi* can gather there.

Chi Kung adjusts your mind and nervous system. Your mind should be relaxed and loose. It will help if you put a happy expression on your face. Become composed. To achieve mental quietness, you need to focus your thoughts and consciousness completely on the exercise itself. In this way, you will be able to keep distracting thoughts and diversions caused by sound and light to a minimum. Of course, it is normal for beginners to become distracted. If this occurs, it may help to suggest mentally to yourself that you need to be patient and that you do have the will to overcome the problem. Mental suggestions such as these will often calm the mind. With persistent practice, your mental concentration will gradually improve. It is not unusual for a Chi Kung exerciser to lose the sensation of body weight temporarily upon entering into a state of mental serenity; at a higher level the practitioner may also lose their sense of self for a while.

THE THREE ASPECTS OF CHI KUNG

Body posture
The spine must be straight and vertical 99 percent of the time so that the *chi* can flow correctly.

Mind and nervous system
When the mind is allowed to become calm, the nervous system will likewise be soothed.

Breathing cycle
Correct breathing generates and circulates *chi* and helps regulate the mind and the emotions.

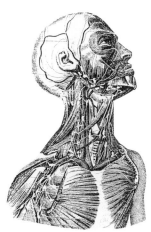

■ The acupuncture meridian system and the nervous system influence each other.

Chi Kung adjusts your respiration or breathing cycle. You need to integrate the training of *yi*—your consciousness—with the training of *chi*, by regulating your respiration. You must learn how to direct the movement of *chi* with your consciousness. In other words, let your thought control your breathing. Let your consciousness adjust the regularity, duration, volume, and speed of your breathing. To condition *yi* is to attain mental quietness. To condition *chi* is to regulate your breathing by following the implications of these seven words: full, deep, long, slow, steady, soft, and even. Through conditioning, you will ultimately be able to lead or follow the movement of *chi* with *yi*.

Chi Kung attempts to achieve a state of mental tranquility and quietness without involving the movement of the body. In order to maintain a proper balance between body movement and mental quietness, you should also engage in other forms of therapeutic exercises. Better therapeutic effects can be achieved when combining Chi Kung with action-orientated exercises, such as Tai Chi. Chi Kung, however, should be performed before the other exercises.

There are various types of Chi Kung. The most popular types today, however—and those described in more detail in this book—are Fang Sung Kung, which is relaxation breathing; Chiang Chuang Kung, invigorating breathing; and Nei Yang Kung, internally nourishing breathing. While Chiang Chuang Kung and Fang Sung Kung place greater emphasis on conditioning *yi*, Nei Yang Kung focuses more on conditioning *chi*. Whatever the method used, all techniques of Chi Kung are designed to integrate *yi* with *chi*.

Regulating the mind, the breath, and *chi* are all equally important and should be practiced and developed together. The three elements are inseparable, for without any one of them we would die. Nourishing all three together prolongs life.

■ Three-circle Chi Kung (*right*) is good for everyone; the weak and infirm can do an easier version (*far right*).

Benefits of Chi Kung

The ancient technique of Chi Kung is the perfect remedy for many modern ills.

✱ Chi Kung inhibits cortical—or thinking brain—activities, so that overstimulated and overworked nerve cells in the cortex can be rejuvenated.

✱ This in turn is very beneficial in the treatment of diseases that are closely related to the condition of the individual's nervous system and mental state, such as depression, anxiety, gastric and duodenal ulcers, and high blood pressure.

✱ Chi Kung helps restore depleted energy reserves, making it especially effective for those who are generally run-down.

✱ The breathing movement of Chi Kung effectively massages the organs inside the abdominal cavity, which can speed up stomach and intestinal movement, reduce abdominal sluggishness, and improve digestion and absorption. For this reason, it is known to be beneficial in treating habitual constipation.

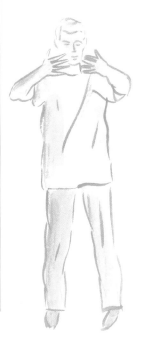

Chi Kung: The Basics

Mastering any new technique takes time and plenty of practice, and Chi Kung is no exception. Although you may experience some initial problems, none of these is difficult to overcome if you follow the advice given here. Remember that it is essential to practice Chi Kung regularly—which means every day—in order to reap all the rewards that it can offer.

BREATHING SHOULD BE COMPLETELY NATURAL—AND NEVER FORCED

SPINE MUST ALWAYS BE STRAIGHT, BUT RELAXED

If properly done, you will not normally have any unexpected reactions as a result of practicing Fang Sung Kung, Chiang Chuang Kung, and Nei Yang Kung. It is not unusual, however, for beginners occasionally to experience certain reactions because they have not yet become accustomed to the new posture, breathing rhythm, and the requirements for mental concentration. Failure to practice the exercise correctly may also lead to problems. In general, abnormal reactions can be prevented or overcome by making necessary adjustments. Some possible problems and ways to handle them are outlined below.

✳ **Postural problems:** If you have soreness and pain in your waist and back, the cause is most often an uncomfortable or inappropriate sitting position. You can overcome this by starting the exercise in the lying-down position and then working up to the sitting position. Or, whenever you feel tired, immediately switch to the lying-down position. Another alternative is simply to reduce the sitting time.

■ **It may take a little while before you are proficient enough to start in the sitting position.**

✳ **Breathing problems:** If you have an unsteady breathing rhythm or if your breathing feels uncomfortable, it is probably due to the beginner's failure to follow the correct breathing procedure because of impatience. Instead of letting your breathing occur naturally, you may have attempted to force it to become deep and long. This problem can be corrected simply by letting your breathing become spontaneous and natural. If you wish, you can walk around indoors for a while to let your emotions calm down before returning to the exercise.

Some beginners experience congestion and a feeling of obstruction in their chest and pain around their ribs. This is most often caused by breathing with too much force or by holding your breath for too long. These sensations may also occur if you stop inhaling at the chest or throat level. You can avoid these abnormal reactions by using the correct method for breathing.

✳ **Problems with mental concentration:** Drowsiness and sleepiness can occur if you are tired and practice Chi Kung in the lying-down position. To overcome this, switch to a sitting position or, alternatively, open your eyes slightly and look at the tip of your nose.

As a rule, it is not a good idea to practice Chi Kung when you are tired. It is quite natural, however, for the beginner sometimes to fall asleep. To prevent drowsiness, you may find it helpful to drink a little hot tea and walk a few steps indoors before engaging in Chi Kung.

ESSENTIALS OF CHI KUNG

◆ As a kung fu, Chi Kung must be practiced every day, following a gradual progression, in order to achieve proficiency. It can not be done overnight.

◆ To develop the proper body posture and to master the breathing techniques, you should begin with the easy ones before attempting to do the more complicated ones.

◆ You should also follow the procedure step by step in order to learn the technique of *ju ching* —entering into a state of mental quietness.

◆ About 10 to 15 minutes before engaging in the exercise, terminate all mental work and eliminate body wastes.

◆ Don't do Chi Kung either right after a meal or on an empty stomach. Nor should you practice Chi Kung when you are suffering from a fever, diarrhea, a bad cold, or are physically tired.

◆ In the beginning, your practice session should be brief, generally no more than 15 or 20 minutes. Later, you can extend the time to 30 minutes.

◆ Set the amount of time for the exercise based on your health, fitness, and mood. After the exercise is over, don't stand up immediately. First rub your face with both hands (see p. 56, set 3) and gently massage your eyes before getting up slowly. Stretch your arms and legs.

◆ If during the exercise you find your breathing rhythm shallow and uneven, you should look for the reasons. The problem is likely to be caused by one of the following: an incorrect method of breathing, a negative frame of mind, lack of desire to do the exercise, or mental distractions. Correct the problem before continuing.

◆ If you get a headache or experience dizziness or a sensation of heaviness in your head, you are probably trying so hard that you are causing an unnatural breathing rhythm. Impatience and emotional agitation may be responsible. Find the cause and correct it.

Sometimes after entering a state of mental quietness, your skin may begin itching or burning, feel as if insects are crawling on it, or feel numb. These sensations are a sign that the deep breathing has successfully mobilized your energy.

❊ **Other symptoms**: Occasionally people experience palpitations: generally these are caused by inhaling or holding the breath for too long, but they may also result from emotional agitation. Correct the problem by maintaining a smooth breathing rhythm and calming your emotions.

If you experience a throbbing sensation in your temporal artery while lying on your side, you can get rid of it by changing the position of your head to take pressure off your ear.

■ **After performing Chi Kung gently massage your face and the area around your eyes.**

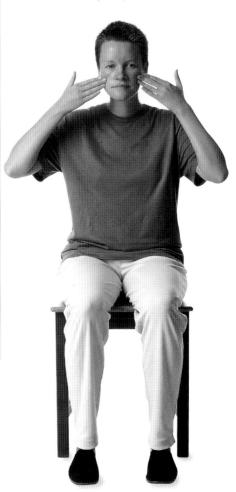

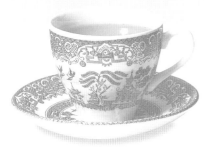

■ **A cup of hot tea may help to alleviate drowsiness, especially when you are practicing Chi Kung lying down.**

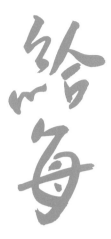

(5)

FANG SUNG KUNG

Relaxation Breathing

Relatively easy to do, Fang Sung Kung can help treat all kinds of chronic diseases, especially respiratory and neurological conditions.

The technique of *ju ching*—entering into mental quietness—involves using certain words to induce relaxation. As you inhale, think of the word "quiet." As you exhale, think of the word "relax." While thinking "relax," consciously let a certain part of your body relax. Relax one part during each breathing cycle. Go from your head to your arms, hands, chest, abdomen, back, waist, buttocks, legs, and, finally, your feet. After the muscles of your entire body have been relaxed, mentally suggest to your blood vessels, nerves, and internal organs that they also relax.

In ancient China poems were used as instructions so that those who were illiterate could remember them. Chinese doctors offer the relaxation poem on the facing page.

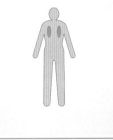

ESSENTIAL POINTS

■ Relax the individual parts of your body one by one, working from the top of the body right down to the soles of the feet.

■ Keep your breathing steady, with the same rhythm and depth that you use for normal, everyday breathing.

1 Begin by lying on your back on the floor. Place a thick pillow or cushion under your head and support your shoulders and back with a towel if necessary.

2 Keep your head straight and your arms extended beside your body. Your legs should be stretched out naturally. Keep your eyes partially closed.

3 Close your mouth naturally and let your upper and lower teeth gently touch each other. The tip of your tongue should touch the roof of your mouth.

4 Breathe naturally in and out through your nose. What is important in Fang Sung Kung is that you regulate your breathing so that it is full, which means it should be soundless; even, which means it has a constant speed and depth; and steady, which means it should be unrestrained and unobstructed. You should do Fang Sung Kung with the same frequency that you do Chiang Chuang Kung (see *p. 77*).

EYES ARE HALF-SHUT

MOUTH IS CLOSED

ARMS LIE RELAXED
ALONGSIDE THE BODY

The Poem of Fang Sung Kung

🌿 🌿 🌿

With a high pillow I lie on my bed;
I keep my body comfortable and relaxed.
I breathe in and out naturally,
And say the words "quiet" and "relax" silently.
I think of the word "quiet" as I inhale,
And the word "relax" as I exhale.
As I silently say the word "relax,"
I tell my muscles to relax.
First, I relax my head, arms, and neck,
Then my chest, abdomen, waist, and back.
Finally, I tell my legs and feet to become relaxed.
After repeating this three times to get my body at ease,
I tell all my organs and cavities to relax.
I keep my breathing rhythm steady, narrow, and even
While focusing my attention on my abdomen.
As my mind enters into a state of mental quietness,
I enjoy this sleeplike but awake state of consciousness.
After staying in this state for a short period of time,
I rub my face, get up, move around, and feel fine.

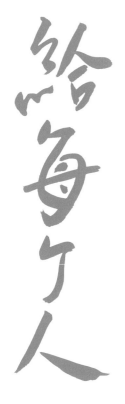

6

CHIANG CHUANG KUNG

Invigorating Breathing

Chiang Chuang Kung can be used to treat diseases such as anxiety and depression, as well as being effective in relieving some of the symptoms of high blood pressure, heart disease, and emphysema. This form of invigorating breathing pays special attention to *ju ching*, the technique of entering into the state of mental quietness, and is not as demanding as some other types of Chi Kung in terms of its requirements for regulating the breathing rhythm.

In this form of Chi Kung, an ordinary sitting position is most often used, but you can also adopt a cross-legged or standing position. The physically weak may use a lying-down position, lying either on the right-hand side of the body or on the back (*see p. 72*). You should always avoid lying on the left-hand side of the body, since the body weight presses on the heart and obstructs its function, thereby impairing the circulation.

The recommended position is sitting straight on a sturdy stool or chair.

1 **Place both feet firmly on the ground, shoulder-width apart.** Your knees should form a 90-degree angle and your body should be straight. Your thighs and trunk should also form a 90-degree angle.

2 **Place your hands, palms down, gently on your legs.** Let your elbows bend naturally. Keep your head, waist and back straight. Let your shoulders fall naturally. Let your chest and chin turn slightly inward. Keep your eyes partially closed. Close your mouth naturally and let your upper and lower teeth gently touch each other. The tip of your tongue should touch the roof of your mouth.

ESSENTIAL POINTS

- Breathe deeply in your abdomen.
- Pause after each exhalation and silently recite a calm-inducing phrase.
- Do not hold your breath or tense your muscles.

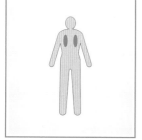

TRUNK AND THIGHS FORM A RIGHT ANGLE

LOWER LEGS AND THIGHS ARE ALSO AT RIGHT ANGLES

SET 1 Holy lotus posture

Sit in the lotus position. **Place one hand on top of the other near your navel or on your abdomen, with your thumbs crossing each other. Keep your eyes partially closed. Close your mouth naturally and let your upper and lower teeth gently touch each other. The tip of your tongue should touch the roof of your mouth.**

SET 2 Cross-legged posture

Alternatively, adopt a natural cross-legged position, with your feet under your legs, your knees off the floor, and your buttocks sticking slightly out behind you. Keep your spine as straight as possible. This lets *chi* rise up the spine along the Governing Meridian. Keep your head and waist straight and your chest curved slightly in. Let your shoulders drop naturally. Place one hand on top of the other on your abdomen, with the thumbs crossing each other.

MOUTH IS CLOSED

MEN PLACE THE LEFT PALM ON THE ABDOMEN WITH THE RIGHT ON TOP; WOMEN THE OPPOSITE

If you prefer a standing position, then the three-circle Chi Kung posture is best, but it is appropriate only for relatively healthy people.

In this position, you can use either natural breathing or abdominal deep breathing. To breathe naturally, just breathe in and out through your nose as described for Fang Sung Kung (*see pp. 72–73*).

With abdominal deep breathing, your abdomen will swell naturally as you inhale, and contract as you exhale. If you wish,

you can place your hands on your abdomen so that you can actually feel the movement (*see below*). You should gradually increase the depth of each inhalation and exhalation until the number of your breathing cycles has been reduced to 6 to 8 per minute. Although the duration of each breathing cycle is lengthened, your breathing must still be natural and relaxed. Never tense your muscles or apply force. Never attempt to breathe deeply through unnatural effort.

ARMS ARE LEVEL WITH
THE SHOULDERS

FEELING THE
MOVEMENT OF
ABDOMINAL
BREATHING

SET 3 ▐ Three-circle Chi Kung posture

Stand with your feet shoulder-width apart, your toes pointing slightly inward and your knees slightly bent. Keep your waist straight, your chest flat, and your arms raised in front of you at about shoulder level, as if you were embracing a large tree. Your elbows may be a bit lower than your shoulders. Bend your fingers as if you were holding an imaginary ball in your hands.

KNEES ARE
FLEXED

1

2

Ju ching, entering mental quietness, is the key here. The fundamental principle of Chiang Chuang Kung is to focus *yi*, your consciousness, on your lower abdomen. In the beginning, you may develop the habit of concentration by silently counting or mentally following the movement of each breathing cycle. With practice, you will eventually learn to focus attention passively on your lower abdomen without effort.

To use the breath-counting method, silently count each time you inhale and exhale. Count from one to ten and then back to one again. If you lose track of the counting because of mental distractions, just start the counting over again. Focusing on your breathing is a more natural method than counting breaths. Let your thoughts gently follow the movement of each breathing rhythm. Keep your attention on your breathing. If distractions occur, recall your thoughts and concentrate once again on the movement of each breath.

The *yi* focusing method—another way of getting mentally quiet—involves thinking of the energy center Tan Tien, which is about 3in (7.5cm) below your navel. The idea is to place your thoughts very gently and easily on this spot without trying, in order to activate the *chi*. Do not force yourself to concentrate. Let it be completely natural. If distractions do occur, return your thoughts to the same spot again.

Chiang Chuang Kung progression chart

	WEEK 1	WEEKS 2 TO 4	WEEK 5 ONWARD
Posture	Lying or sitting on chair	Sitting on chair or cross-legged	Sitting or standing position
Breathing	Natural breathing progressing to moderate deep breathing	Abdominal deep breathing	Abdominal deep breathing
Consciousness	Counting breaths; following breaths	Following breaths; placing *yi* on lower abdomen	Placing *yi* on the lower abdomen
Frequency and duration	3 to 4 times daily 15 to 20 minutes a time	3 to 4 times daily 30 minutes a time	3 to 4 times daily 30 to 40 minutes a time
Essentials	▲ Correct posture ▲ Breathing is deep, even, and steady but with latent energy ▲ Eliminate mental distractions	▲ Longer and deeper breathing, *chi* sinking into Tan Tien ▲ Initial mental quietness ▲ Regular practice	▲ Breathing is now steady, deep, long, slow, soft and even ▲ Complete mental quietness, or *ju ching* ▲ Interest in Chi Kung

給每个人

(7)

NEI YANG KUNG

Internally Nourishing Breathing

If you are generally run-down or suffering from abdominal disorders, including ulcers or habitual constipation, Nei Yang Kung is especially valuable. It pays special attention to the technique of breathing itself. The best positions for this exercise are lying on your side and regular sitting as for Chiang Chuang Kung (*see pp. 74–75*), but you can also lie on your back as for Fang Sung Kung (*see pp. 72–73*).

Using the correct breathing method, which involves some new techniques, is especially important with this Chi Kung. Begin by breathing in and out through your nose, using the abdominal method (*see pp. 76–77*). Then pause for a moment between each breathing cycle. More specifically, inhale and exhale, pause and raise your tongue to the roof of your mouth, and silently recite a few words before lowering your tongue and inhaling. The phrase or sentence you

SET 1 | Reclining *chi* posture

Lie on your right-hand side with your head on a pillow and bent slightly forward. Bend your right arm beside your chest and place your hand on the pillow about 2in (5cm) away from your head with your palm up. Stretch your left arm out naturally and place your hand on your hip, palm down. Bend both legs naturally, with your left leg on top of your right, or use any position that feels natural and relaxing.

ESSENTIAL POINTS

- Breathe deeply in your abdomen.
- Pause after each exhalation and silently recite a calm-inducing phrase.
- Do not hold your breath or tense your muscles.

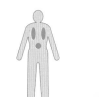

RIGHT PALM FACES UPWARD,
BESIDE THE HEAD

LEFT ARM RELAXES ON TOP OF THE BODY

choose should have an appropriate message, for example, "Be peaceful," "Good to be peaceful" or "Relaxation is good for health."

During the moment that you pause, do not tense your muscles and hold your breath. Nor should you stop the breath in your upper abdomen or throat. In a breathing pause, the aim is to center your consciousness on the lower abdomen, with a temporary halt in breathing. The duration of the pause may be gradually increased as you recite more words. It takes about a second to recite one word; most people recite between three and seven words. By coordinating your breathing with the silent recitation of a phrase or sentence, your concentration is guided and you will gradually enter *ju ching*, the state of mental quietness. The physiological effects of breathing pause need further study, but it appears that this type of breathing tends to create pressure in the abdominal cavity, which results in improved blood circulation and intestinal movement, and significantly increases the transformation of energy.

SET 2 ‖ Holy lotus posture

Sit in the lotus position with the spine vertical and straight. Keep the shoulders totally relaxed and the face at ease, wearing a slight smile. In this way the *chi* that is generated will have a positive nature.

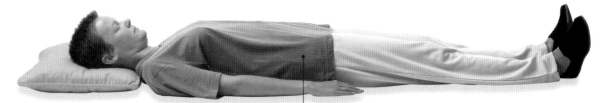

SET 3 ‖ Lying-down *chi* posture

Stretch out full length on the floor with a pillow or cushion under your head. Totally relax your body and let the ground support you. Imagine that you are bathed in warm sunlight, at peace with yourself and with the natural world around you.

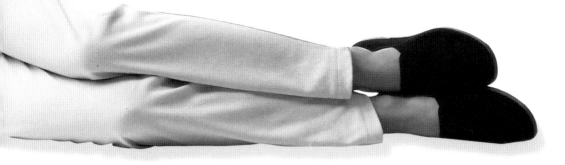

BODY IS TOTALLY AT EASE

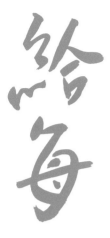

8

SHEN HU XI YUN DONG

Up and Down Gymnastic
Breathing Exercise

Although easy to do, this breathing exercise can help develop your overall fitness. Involving the movement of the entire body and coordination between motion and breathing, this up-and-down exercise series must be done slowly and softly, with a long, even breathing rhythm.

ESSENTIAL POINTS

- Breathe in as you move upward and lift your arms.
- Breathe out as you squat and lower your arms.
- Keep your upper body straight at all times.

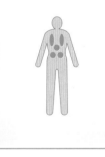

● *This exercise speeds up blood circulation and the digestion of food, improves the ability to take in air, absorb oxygen, and expel carbon dioxide, and strengthens both the chest and the abdominal muscles, particularly the breathing muscles.*

Relax your entire body. Stand naturally with your feet shoulder-width apart and your arms hanging quite naturally. Mentally concentrate on the movements as you do them slowly and evenly. Breathe quite naturally.

ARMS ARE SLOWLY LOWERED AS YOU SQUAT DOWN

2 **With your arms just** slightly bent and your fingers curled naturally, lift your hands over your head from the front. At the same time, breathe in. Begin inhaling as you start to lift your hands and finish inhaling when your hands are over your head.

I

2

3a

3 Next bend both knees, open your hands, lower your arms, and start to squat down.

3b

4 Keep your upper body straight and lower your arms to the front as you squat down naturally, while exhaling. Note that squatting, arm lowering, and exhaling all start and finish at the same time. Once you are at ground level and your hands have been fully lowered, place them beside your legs.

4

5 Then rise up on your legs again as you simultaneously lift your arms to the front and over your head. As you do this, breathe in. Count each up-and-down movement cycle as one exercise. You may repeat it 10 to 20 times, depending on your state of health, but avoid excessive repetitions as they may cause dizziness. If the number of repetitions is about right, you should feel refreshed after completing the exercise.

5

6 Once you are quite proficient at doing this movement, you may also rotate your body from side to side while you are in the standing position. Turn your whole body, including head and neck, to the left and then the right. This rotation should be done when you are in the standing position, with your arms raised. You should exhale as you do it.

6

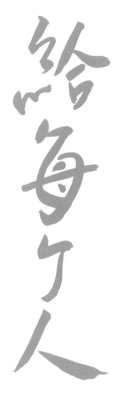

9

TAI JI GUN

Tai Chi Rod

One of many ancient Chinese fitness methods, Tai Chi Rod is basically the same as Tai Chi in terms of its demand for relaxation, peacefulness, and spontaneity. It, too, integrates movement with mental quietness and, because it uses a rod 12in (30cm) long, is called Tai Chi Rod or Tai Chi Ruler. (It does not matter whether the rod is thick or thin, but it must be wooden.)

The exercise is simple to do and can be performed either sitting or standing. The physically weak or sick may even do it lying down. The only movement it requires is to circle your hands in front of your chest or to move them up and down. Before you start the exercise, open the window to let some fresh air in and make sure the environment is quiet.

Relax your entire body. Close your eyes partially and breathe naturally. Focus *yi*, or consciousness, on your lower abdomen. Just lie, sit, or

ESSENTIAL POINTS

- The movements must be soft and slow, comfortable and natural.
- Increase exercise length and frequency gradually— do not try to accomplish everything in one day.

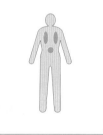

SET 1 | Sitting position
In the sitting position, you can use any posture that is comfortable. With your palms against the ends of the rod as described, bend your elbows and draw circles in front of your abdomen.

SET 2 | Standing position
To do the exercise standing up, you should keep your feet shoulder-width apart. Then, again holding the rod as described, draw circles in front of your abdomen.

CAUTION

Do not do this exercise if you are suffering from any acute disease, fever, or bleeding.

stand and relax quietly for a little while. Then press your palms against the ends of the rod, hold it in front of your abdomen, and move both your hands in front of your abdomen as if you were turning a wheel.

Practice time is usually set at 2 to 5 minutes in the beginning. After 20 to 30 days, you may increase the practice time to 5 to 10 minutes. After another 1 to 2 months, you may increase it to 10 to 20 minutes. Do not increase the time after this. You may practice Tai Chi Rod 2 to 3 times a day.

After doing Tai Chi Rod for a while, it is possible you may experience a few abnormal reactions. You may feel heat and perspiration throughout your body, you may itch, your fingers may swell, or your muscles may twitch. The reactions are similar to those that may be experienced when performing Chi Kung (see pp. 70–71). The movements of Tai Chi Rod will also accelerate stomach and intestinal movement: you may hear noises coming from your intestines and feel the urge to break wind. You may also find your appetite significantly improved.

SET 4 ∥ Walking position

Once you have improved your physical strength, you may add to these exercises, drawing circles while walking or walking on the spot. To draw circles with the rod while walking on the spot, stand with one foot in front and one foot behind. Lift one foot up and replace it on the same spot. Then do the same with the other foot. When the foot is up, draw one circle with the rod. When the foot is down, also draw one circle with the rod. Alternate which foot comes in front. When drawing circles while walking, you should draw one circle for each step taken. Be sure to keep your knees slightly bent at all times.

SET 3 ∥ Lying position

When performing the exercise while lying on your back, bend your elbows and keep them on the bed or floor at all times during the exercise. The motion involves pressing your palms against the ends of the rod and swaying the rod up and down in a continuous movement.

75%

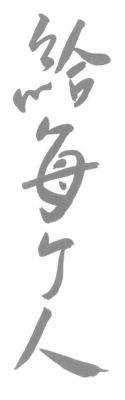

10

TSA FU PEI

Knocking at the Gate of Life

The ancient fitness method of Tsa Fu Pei literally means to knock the abdomen and back, and combines massage, knocking, and waist exercise. It is effective and easy to do, and it can be performed anywhere.

According to traditional Chinese medicine, the area located 3in (7.5cm) below the navel is called Tan Tien. It is so important that it has the alternative name of Chien Ming Men (The Front Gate of Life). The corresponding position on the back is Ming Men (Life Gate) or Hau Ming Men (The Back Gate of Life). Because this exercise involves knocking in the vicinity of the Ming Men acupuncture points (the one on the back is below the second lumbar vertebra on the Governing

ESSENTIAL POINTS

- To create the natural force of the knocking, you should loosen your entire body and rely on your waist as the axis of the rotation.
- Pay special attention to relaxing your arms.
- Keep your breathing natural. You may breathe only through your nose or through both your nose and mouth at the same time.

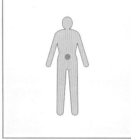

1 | Relax your entire body. Now bend your knees slightly and make loose fists. Let your arms hang down naturally. Focus *yi*, or consciousness, on your navel.

2 Start by placing your loose fists against your front and back life gates. Then turn your body at the waist to start your arms swinging. Let your left loose fist strike just below your navel as the right one hits the Ming Men region of your back.

1

2

Meridian), it is also called Knocking at the Gate of Life.

The best time to do Tsa Fu Pei is in the morning when there is plenty of fresh air. Do not exercise immediately after a meal—wait at least an hour after eating. The knocking will vibrate your internal organs and help improve your digestion and speed up blood circulation.

The real center of the body's energy is located halfway between Chien Ming Men, or the Front Gate of Life, on the front of the body and the Ming Men point on the back. The front and back points are themselves just access points. The actual energy center is the True Tan Tien—Tan Tien meaning "Field of the Elixir" (as in "the elixir of life"). We always try to assimilate more *chi* in our True Tan Tien in order to increase our longevity and vitality.

3 Then let your right fist knock your front and the left fist your back. While turning at the waist to the left and right, your arms should swing like ropes, without the slightest effort, and your hands and fists should act like hammers. The knocking should be induced by the natural force of your turning motion, not by the stiff force of your arms. You can adjust the frequency and duration of the knocking according to your needs—if the exercise load is about right, you should feel relaxed and comfortable and perspire a little. Apply force progressively, however. Do not overreach yourself by increasing the exercise load too fast.

3

⑪

LI SHOU

Hand Swinging

This exercise, with its simple and easy movement, has been passed down from generation to generation in China. It is well known for its effectiveness in increasing physical strength and building up resistance to disease, and is especially suitable for the elderly and physically weak, as well as for patients with chronic diseases in general. You can vary the number of swings per session and the number of sessions per day to suit yourself and your condition.

When practicing Li Shou, you need to maintain a comfortable and natural posture, keep your movements loose and follow the correct method persistently. As with other fitness methods, you should proceed step by step, increasing the number of swings you do only gradually. You should not get

> Keep your spine relaxed but upright, your chest straight but comfortable. Do not thrust your chest forward. Keep your waist and stomach loose. Don't stick your stomach out. If you are doing this correctly, you will naturally feel heavy and full in the abdomen.

the idea that the more you swing, the better. In fact, swinging for too long may do more harm than good.

Li Shou has evolved into more than ten variations. The following is one of the most fundamental and popular varieties, known to have among the best healing effects.

Keep your neck loose and your face natural throughout the exercise. Put on a happy face—it will help you become relaxed. Close your mouth and let your lips and teeth gently touch. Let your tongue lie flat. Loosen your clothes and belt. Begin by standing with your feet shoulder-width apart. Keep your body straight and let your arms hang down naturally by your side. Look straight ahead of you. Make sure that you feel quite comfortable. Place your toes, soles, and heels firmly and evenly on the ground, with your toes pointing forward.

SPINE IS STRAIGHT AND STOMACH LOOSE

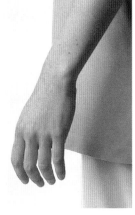

Once the hands are swinging, the fingers should be slightly parted, with the palms facing inward and slightly bent.

1

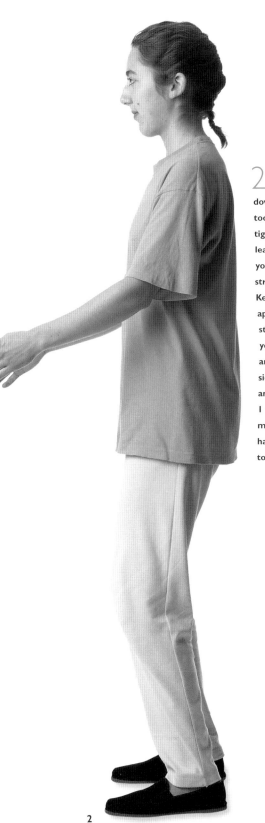

2 **Keep your shoulders loose and let them hang down. Let your arms hang, too, and do not hold them tightly against your body— leave some space under your armpits. Don't straighten your elbows. Keep your fingers naturally apart—do not bend or straighten them. Keep your palms slightly bent and facing toward your sides. Now relax your body and calm your mind for 1 to 2 minutes. Then you may start swinging your hands fluidly from front to back.**

3 **When your arms are out in front your thumbs should not be higher than the navel. When your hands are being swung back, the outer edges of your little fingers should not move higher than your buttocks.**

HANDS GO NO
HIGHER THAN
THE BUTTOCKS

2

3

ESSENTIALS OF LI SHOU

◆ Whenever possible, perform Li Shou in clean air and a quiet environment. Stop practicing if there is a thunderstorm, because the electrical activity in the atmosphere could interfere with the smooth flow of *chi* through the body.

◆ Avoid doing Li Shou right after a heavy meal or when hungry.

◆ Your entire body must be relaxed, particularly your shoulders, arms, and hands. Relaxation will facilitate the circulation of *chi* and blood, causing them both to flow downward. This way your lower body will become heavy and firm. While swinging your hands, you should have a feeling that is known in China as empty-top-but-solid-bottom.

◆ Your hand swing should be accompanied by the movement of your waist and legs. Do not just swing your arms. Waist movement can help to strengthen your internal organs and thus produce greater effects.

◆ Your breathing should be natural. Do not deliberately attempt to coordinate your hand movements with your breathing rhythm. Greater benefits can be obtained when you learn gradually to breathe with your abdomen.

◆ Your arms should be as loose as a rope. Your fingers should be separated naturally. Do not tense your muscles.

◆ You should integrate external movement and mental quietness. When the two are fully coordinated, the external movement becomes spontaneous. The result is that you will feel good about your entire body.

◆ If you find excess saliva in your mouth, swallow it rather than spitting it out.

◆ Count each back-and-forth swing as one movement. The number of movements differs from person to person, but must be increased only gradually. Do not force yourself to break your own record. As you are swinging your hands, silently count the number of swings. If you prefer, you can swing for a set amount of time.

◆ Keep your eyes partially closed. Keep your mental focus on your navel.

◆ When you are doing Li Shou correctly, you should feel relaxed and comfortable both during and after the exercise.

◆ If you experience any dizziness, chest pain, nausea, or extreme fatigue, you should reduce the number of sessions or stop the exercise for the time being. These problems are most often caused by swinging too many times and swinging with too much force, that is, above the navel in front or higher than the buttocks behind.

◆ After the exercise, remain standing for 1 to 2 minutes. Then do some relaxing exercises before returning to normal activities.

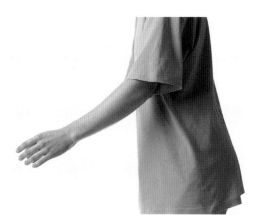

Swinging your hands should be allied to moving your waist slightly—it is not a question of doing one activity at the expense of the other.

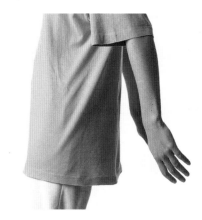

Keep your fingers slightly splayed and make sure that you do not swing them too high—either in front of or behind the body—or overenthusiastically.

During the hand swinging, it is possible that you may feel cold or warm, hear noises coming from your abdomen, or feel the urge to break wind. You may also experience numbness, a swelling pain, or the sensation of insects crawling on your skin. Some people feel the *chi* circulating inside their body; others make involuntary movements. These are normal, but by no means universal, physiological phenomena brought about by the integration of motion with mental quietness

Such happenings are similar to those that may be experienced while practicing Chi Kung. You should not be overly concerned about them, just let them be. Equally, do not make a conscious attempt to produce these reactions.

The gentle arm swinging with a slight waist rotation is beneficial for general health and relaxation. All the internal organs are lightly massaged, the circulation of blood and *chi* is invigorated, and a sense of well-being ensues.

Sitting position

You can also do Li Shou from a sitting position, although you will not get the same waist movements. Sit upright, with your thighs almost at right angles to your lower legs, relax your shoulders, and swing the arms as described for the standing position.

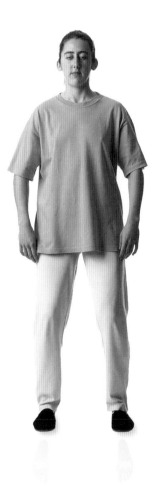

Once you have finished hand swinging, stand perfectly still for a couple of minutes, before doing some gentle exercises to relax yourself.

HANDS SWING
BACK TO THE LEVEL
OF THE THIGHS

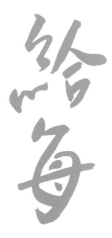

12

YAN BU YUN DONG

Eye Exercises

The use of eye exercises and self-massage to protect the eyesight was widespread in ancient China. According to historical accounts, the most common techniques were:

▶ Turning the eyeballs to the left and then to the right 7 times, closing the eyes tightly for a while, then suddenly opening them wide.

▶ Pressing the center of the small indentation that lies just under the middle of the center of the eyebrow 27 times. Pressing the same concavity with the joint of the thumb 36 times.

▶ Pressing the spot between the inner corner of the eye and the bridge of the nose 36 times.

In recent years, a number of new eye-protection exercises have been developed in China based on the idea that near-sightedness in adolescents is often a result of the improper use of the eyes. For instance, the habit of holding reading material too close to the eyes can cause eyestrain, or it can trigger spasmodic contractions in the eyelid muscles. As a result, the lens of the eye may thicken because it is temporarily pulled out of shape. This kind of near-sightedness is called pseudo-near-sightedness, because the refraction angles have not yet been permanently lengthened, and eye-protection exercises can often be beneficial for this condition. Massaging the acupuncture points around the eyes can help prevent near-sightedness because it improves the adaptability of the eye muscles, reduces spasm, and improves the circulation.

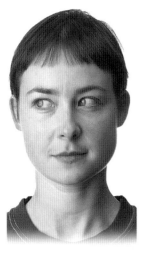

Rolling the eyeballs alternately to left and right 7 times, then closing and opening the eyes suddenly was an ancient Chinese therapy.

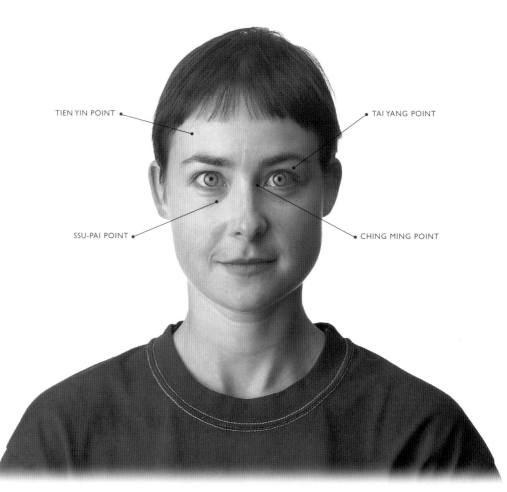

TIEN YIN POINT

TAI YANG POINT

SSU-PAI POINT

CHING MING POINT

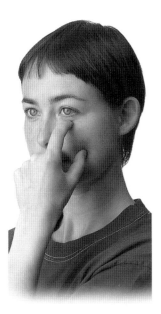

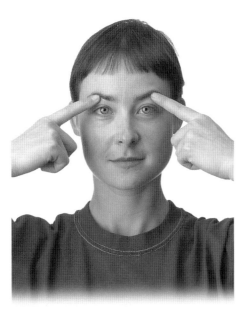

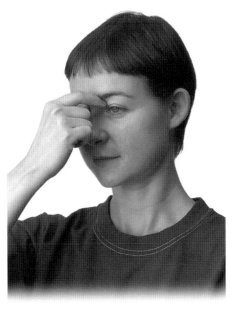

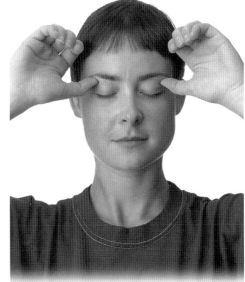

Knead the Ssu-Pai point. First, press your index and middle fingers together, then place them on the side of the bridge of your nose. Your thumb will naturally fit against your lower cheekbone. Without removing your thumb from your cheek, let your index finger find the spot on the bone right below the lowest portion of your eye socket. Curl your other fingers out of the way and knead the area gently.

Curl your index finger and use the side of the second joint to rub all the way around your eye socket, beginning at the top near your nose. By doing this, you massage several acupuncture points, such as Tsan-Chu, Yu-Yao, Ssu-Chu-Kang, Tung-Tzu-Chiao, and Cheng-Chi at the same time.

Gently rub with your thumb the Tien Yin acupuncture point, which lies between the eyebrow and the upper corner of the orbital cavity—the bony structure that surrounds the eye.

Use your thumb and index finger to press and squeeze the Ching Ming points, which lie just beyond the inner corner of the eye on the nose. First press downward, then squeeze upward.

Use your thumb to rub the Tai Yang point in the hollow right below the end of your eyebrow.

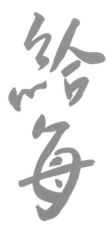

ESSENTIAL POINTS

■ For best results combine dietary supplementation with breathing techniques and hair-loss exercises.

(13)

TUO FA

Hair Loss

The reasons for baldness are quite complicated. It may be related to heredity, anemia, iron deficiency, drugs, chemotherapy, auto-immune disease or an auto-immune reaction, or general deterioration of health. No satisfactory treatment has yet been found for hair loss, but certain Chinese practices have been found to be helpful in preventing hair loss caused by health-related problems.

Some ancient Chinese medical practitioners suggested that scalp massage could prevent baldness and delay the graying of hair. Modern medicine says that massaging the scalp can indeed stimulate hair follicles and promote normal hair growth. Massage can also remove sebum or dandruff-forming oil and sloughed-off skin cells and their unhealthy effects.

For hair loss, you can also practice Chiang Chuang Kung, or invigorating breathing (*see pp. 74–77*), or Nei Yang Kung, or internally nourishing breathing (*see pp. 78–79*).

Some people, as a result of applying massage and Chi Kung, have undoubtedly reversed the trend toward hair loss. In some individuals, new hair was found on the previously bald spot. You can expect better results if you pay attention to your diet as well as using the techniques described here. People who have anemia and iron deficiency should try vitamin B_{12}, folic acid, and iron supplements. They should also consult their doctor. Chinese doctors recommend that those who have excessive sebum, which is a greasy secretion, on their scalp should try vitamin B_6 and cystine.

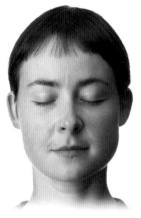

In the distant past a sage introduced an "upward focusing" method for preventing gray hair. While practicing Chi Kung, mentally focus on nothing but the Pai-Hui point. Because the mind goes to the top of the head, so will the *chi*; the blood follows the *chi*, so the roots of the hair will be nourished.

THE PAI-HUI POINT IS LOCATED IN THE EXACT MIDDLE OF THE FLAT PART AT THE TOP OF THE HEAD

TAPPING, RUBBING, AND PULLING TECHNIQUES MAY ALL HELP

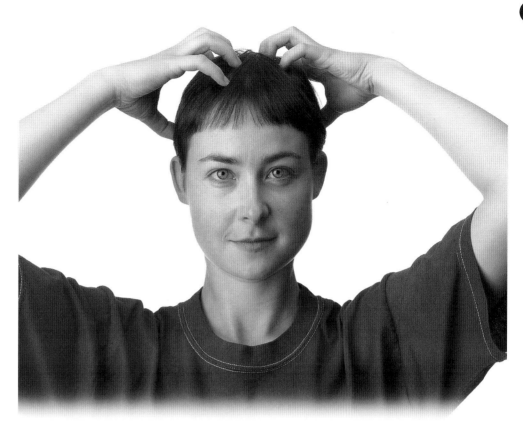

Use your finger tips in the pointing and rapping method
to tap and rap every spot on your head 50 to 100 times.

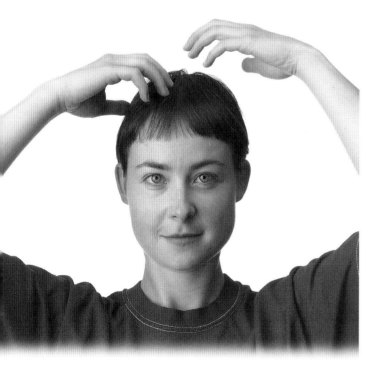

2 Next, rub and knead your scalp with your
fingertips 50 to 100 times.

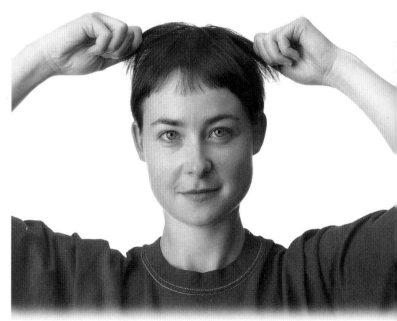

3 Hold a small bunch of your hair between your thumb and index
finger in each hand and gently pull it downward swiftly but
carefully. Do this 20 to 30 times with each clump.

CHAPTER THREE

Combating heart and circulatory disease through healing exercise

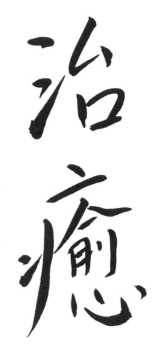

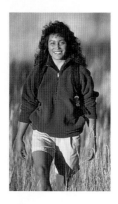

■ **Walking in the open air is one of the best ways to counteract heart disease.**

Heart disease, circulatory disease, and arterial disease are on the increase. They may seem to be different conditions, but they are all connected and have many similar causative factors. The first thing to consider is the composition of the blood— you are what you eat, so a healthy diet will make healthy blood, which will in turn nourish both the heart muscle and the walls of the arteries. If you eat a lot of deep-fried fatty food, then your blood will coagulate and the walls of the arteries will harden and thicken, leading to disease and possibly thrombosis. For the blood to circulate smoothly you should avoid fatty foods and eat lots of fruit and vegetables.

Exercise and correct breathing have a considerable role to play, too. Tai Chi, walking, and many other sports all help to mobilize the blood and *chi* to ensure vigorous, healthy circulation. More than a century ago a doctor developed a form of therapy called pace-determined walking and this represents just one of the routines that can help those with heart disease.

■ The elderly are most susceptible to heart disease, but exercise can help alleviate it.

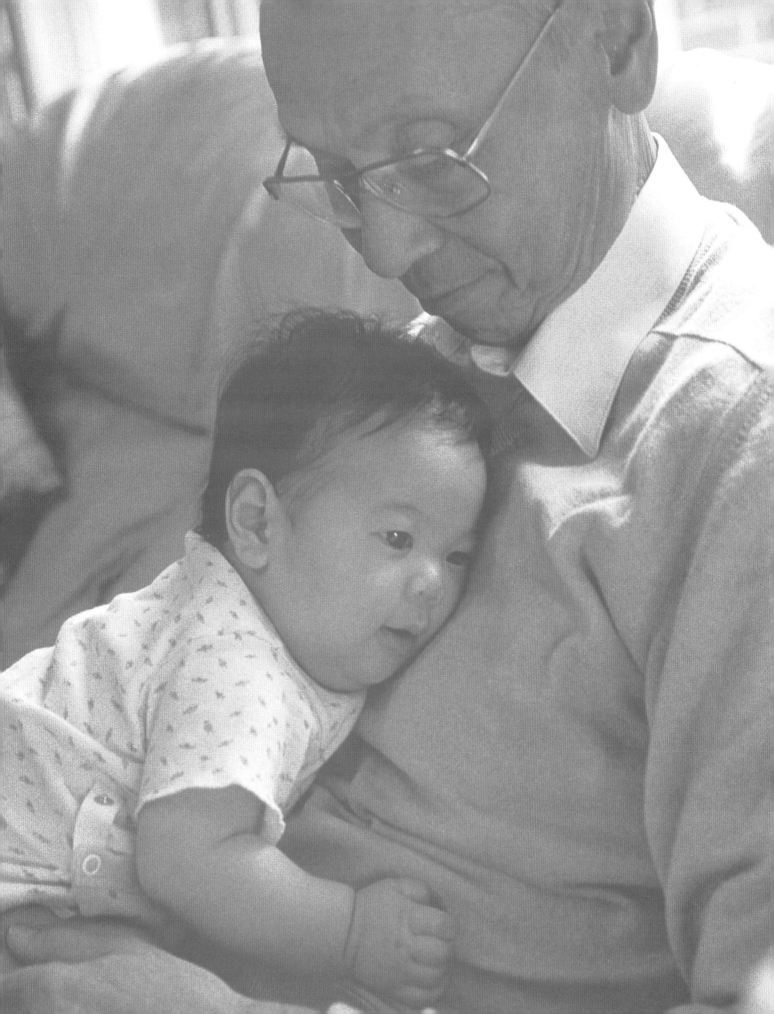

Who Should and Should Not Exercise

We are at a fortunate point in history when we have access to both ancient Chinese medical theory and modern medical techniques, old healing methods and new therapeutic exercises, to help us prevent disease occurring and aid recovery from illness. There is always a self-healing technique for the individual who is keen to take a positive role in improving his or her own health.

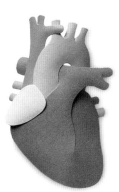

■ The heart is a complex organ and is subject to various different forms of malfunctioning.

Before making any suggestions about exercise for heart patients, it is necessary to issue an extreme caution. Whether or not a heart patient should do healing exercise is a decision that must be made with great care and with the approval of a doctor. Incorrect exercise may do more harm than good, and there is always the possibility that exercise may strain rather than strengthen the heart. Nevertheless, some heart patients unquestionably can better their health and their hearts with healing exercise. If the decision is made to proceed, the patient should seek continued guidance and supervision of the exercise program from his or her doctor.

It is always a good idea to consult a doctor before embarking on an exercise program, but it is essential if any of the following apply: you have any history of coronary artery disease; you are at risk for coronary artery disease because of a history of smoking, elevated cholesterol, or a family history of heart disease; or you are a man over the age of 35 or a woman over 40, who has had a sedentary lifestyle.

The types of exercises that are suitable for patients who have various kinds of heart disease differ according to the patient and his or her condition. A general guide is outlined below; the rest of the chapter deals with specific exercises and their benefits.

✳ **Valvular disease:** Frequently characterized by narrowing and incomplete closing of the mitral or aortic valves in the heart, this condition may rule out team sports, but not necessarily therapeutic exercises. If the circulation is good, pace-determined walking (*see pp. 100–101*), Tai Chi (*see pp. 60–67*), badminton, table tennis, and simple physical fitness exercises may all be appropriate for those who are suffering from valvular disease.

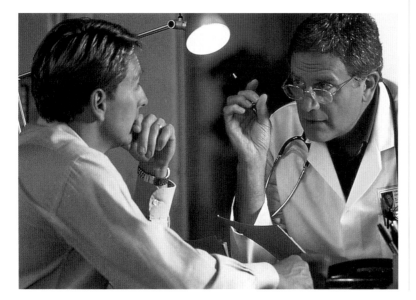

■ Patients with heart or coronary disease should always seek a detailed consultation with their doctor before embarking on any kind of exercise routine.

■ Table tennis is surprisingly energetic and a good form of exercise, as long as it is not taken too seriously.

※ **Congenital heart disease**: This condition, which includes abnormalities of the valves and defects in the heart wall or great vessels, is usually diagnosed in infancy, but may be discovered during physical exercise. Symptoms include fatigue, difficulty in breathing, and change in facial color. Some young people with this disease should do only slow-paced relaxation exercises such as leisurely walking and Tai Chi . They should not engage in team sports, even when their symptoms seem mild. Many can, however, participate in rigorous non-competitive exercise programs. If you have this problem, talk to your doctor about what's right for you.

※ **Functional heart disease**: This category includes people who display disturbances in the nervous system rather than defects in the heart itself. They may find it difficult to perform tasks requiring physical strength. They may feel fatigued, become breathless quickly, and experience pain in the heart region when they exercise. The heart rate at rest may exceed 90 beats per minute (60 to 80, on average, is more normal) and may occasionally be irregular. Patients with this syndrome tend to be irritable and have problems sleeping at night. They should not participate in exercises requiring swift movements. Instead, they should do simple, slow-paced exercises such as walking and Tai Chi.

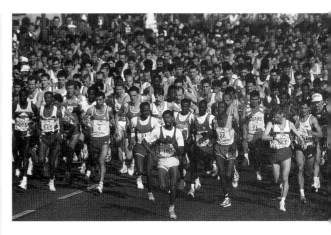

■ Building up stamina by running may be suitable for some people with congenital heart disease.

※ **Arrhythmia:** This is a disturbance in the rhythm of the heart, most commonly extra systole, a premature contraction. If it is caused by organic disease, the patient may have to avoid regular exercise. But someone who occasionally experiences extra systole may exercise under close observation from a health professional.

※ **Coronary heart disease**: People who suffer from the most serious heart diseases, such as myocardial infarction (heart attack) in the acute stage, recurring angina pectoris (acute pain in the heart region), worsening valvular disease, or cardiomyopathy (serious degeneration of the heart muscle) should not do exercises.

■ Tai Chi is gentle enough to be suitable for many people suffering from heart disease.

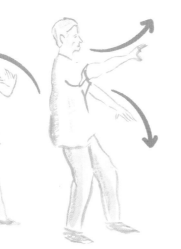

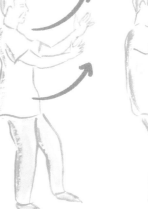

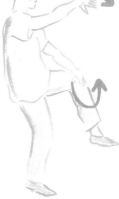

Precautions for Exercising Heart Patients

Care is essential for all those with any form of illness who undertake an exercise program, but this is particularly true for those suffering from heart disease. However, a few simple precautions and careful monitoring can make exercise quite safe and can ensure that heart patients receive all the benefits without having to worry about the risks.

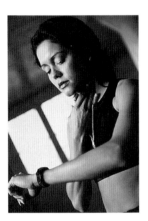

■ **Regular pulse-taking will ensure that you are constantly aware of how much stress your body is under.**

First and foremost, heart patients should take great care not to overburden the hearts they are working to heal. By being careful, the maximum benefits can be obtained from an exercise program. The amount and type of exercise should be chosen, in conjunction with a doctor, based on the condition of the heart.

Before, during, and after exercise, heart patients should carefully monitor their pulse rate and physical reactions. You should never start a workout if your resting heart rate exceeds 90 beats per minute. But it is normal for the pulse rate to increase by 20 or 30 beats per minute immediately after exercise, so this need not be a cause for concern. However, shortness of breath, wheezing, heart palpitations, heart pain, or an irregular heart rhythm are all signals to stop exercising immediately.

Patients who have a fever should not exercise as this can put the heart under increased strain. For every 1.8°F (1°C) increase in body temperature, the heart beats an extra 10 to 20 times a minute, before exercise has even begun.

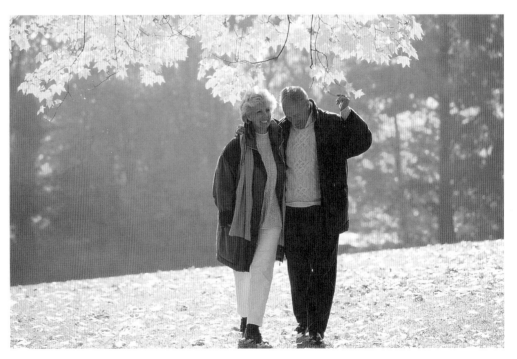

■ **Walking is an ideal form of exercise for most heart patients and also gets them out in the fresh air.**

Categories of heart patients

Exercises intended for chronic heart patients can be divided into four categories, depending on the severity of the disease.

GROUP A

This group of patients is physically weak compared to healthy people, although they can perform their daily chores. However, they can not climb stairs or run as well as the healthy can.

GROUP B

These patients are able to walk slowly on level ground for about 30 minutes without experiencing shortness of breath. But they can not walk fast or climb more than a few stairs.

Patients in categories A and B can enhance their blood circulation and increase the resilience of their heart with well-planned exercises. The heart's ability to perform its task can be improved, and the more it improves, the more it can benefit from a careful exercise program. The basic form of healing exercise should be pace-determined walking (*see pp. 100–101*).

GROUP C

These patients are able to walk slowly for a few hundred steps, but the household routine is a strain. Even breathing may be difficult at times.

GROUP D

Patients in this group are in a critical stage of heart failure, in which cardiac function is so impaired that fluid builds up in the lungs, and breathing is difficult.

Patients in groups C and D can achieve only minor therapeutic effects from exercise. Under the supervision of a doctor, they should choose routines to protect the heart rather than to strengthen it. The most appropriate exercises for them are Chi Kung (*see pp. 68–71*), simplified Tai Chi (*see pp. 60–67*), and walking for pleasure. Exercises are appropriate if they do not excessively speed up the pulse or in any way strain the heart.

GROUP A

GROUP B

GROUP C

GROUP D

Pace-Determined Walking Program

To gain the maximum benefit from walking exercise you should be outdoors in the fresh air of a park or the countryside. Seeing trees, plants, and natural beauty is very healing for the spirit and, since the heart is affected by the mind and the emotions, pleasant surroundings will increase the benefits of walking for those who are recuperating from heart conditions.

The advantage of pace-determined walking is that it can be done anywhere, preferably where there is little traffic and a peaceful atmosphere, perhaps in a park or along quiet streets. The idea behind it is that it is structured in terms of the distance traveled, the speed of walking, and the incline. There are also mandatory rest periods.

All you need is a watch with a second hand or a stopwatch, to time yourself, and some means of measuring out certain distances. You could use a tape measure—for the shorter distances—or a pedometer, which is available from sports stores. Alternatively, once you are walking farther, you could drive the required distance in the car to mark out a walking route.

To begin with, you should walk on level ground and cover a distance of no more than 300yd (300m). Gradually, you will increase this distance to 500yd (500m) —just over quarter of a mile (nearly 0.5km)—then, 1000yd, 1500yd, and 2000yd, (1000m, 1500m, and 2000m) or more, depending on your condition. Walk slowly initially—60 to 80 steps per minute—and take several breaks. As you progress, increase the speed to 80 to 100 steps per minute. Patients who are fitter may walk on very gentle slopes of 3 to 5 degrees for a short distance.

If both weather and health permit, pace-determined walking may be done every other day or even daily. When practiced carefully and consistently, according to the program given opposite, this type of walking may help those who are recuperating from infectious diseases, from chronic heart diseases and from obesity-related heart disease.

The following five-month walking program has been specifically designed for heart patients. Begin with the first month, even if you feel that you could actually manage to do more straight away. Generally speaking, you should stay on each level for a whole month and be able to perform it quite easily before you move on to a higher level. Of course, it is not necessary to adhere rigidly to the recommended distance and speed if it ever feels uncomfortable to do so. But heart patients generally adjust extremely well to this type of pace-determined walking exercise if they follow it systematically.

■ **Walking can be measured, paced, and increased to suit the individual's particular heart condition.**

Five-month walking program

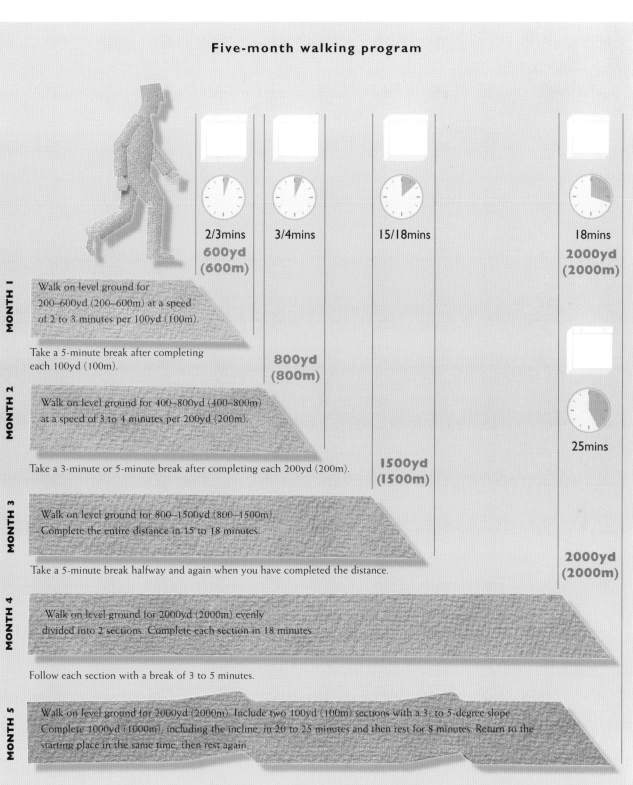

2/3mins
600yd (600m)

3/4mins

15/18mins

18mins
2000yd (2000m)

800yd (800m)

25mins

1500yd (1500m)

2000yd (2000m)

MONTH 1

Walk on level ground for 200–600yd (200–600m) at a speed of 2 to 3 minutes per 100yd (100m).

Take a 5-minute break after completing each 100yd (100m).

MONTH 2

Walk on level ground for 400–800yd (400–800m) at a speed of 3 to 4 minutes per 200yd (200m).

Take a 3-minute or 5-minute break after completing each 200yd (200m).

MONTH 3

Walk on level ground for 800–1500yd (800–1500m). Complete the entire distance in 15 to 18 minutes.

Take a 5-minute break halfway and again when you have completed the distance.

MONTH 4

Walk on level ground for 2000yd (2000m) evenly divided into 2 sections. Complete each section in 18 minutes.

Follow each section with a break of 3 to 5 minutes.

MONTH 5

Walk on level ground for 2000yd (2000m). Include two 100yd (100m) sections with a 3- to 5-degree slope. Complete 1000yd (1000m), including the incline, in 20 to 25 minutes and then rest for 8 minutes. Return to the starting place in the same time, then rest again.

Follow each section with a break of 8 minutes.

■ For the purposes of this book, 1yd=1m throughout

Breathing Exercises and the Heart Patient

Emotion is linked to the heart and people suffering from a broken heart due to emotional stress can actually experience physical problems with this body organ, while mental tension causes physical tension, which in turn impedes blood flow. For these reasons Chi Kung to relax the mind and calm the emotions can also be highly beneficial for the heart.

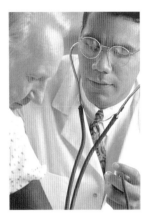

Medical practitioners in China in recent years have used Chi Kung—the classic breathing exercises—to treat heart disease with highly successful results. The therapeutic effects of Chi Kung on the heart include relief from heart palpitations, improved breathing, diminution of dizziness, and an increase in energy. You will be able to relax and sleep better. Your appetite will improve and you will not tire as easily. To get these results, be sure to breathe naturally, freely, and without tension when practicing Chi Kung. Tense, unnatural breathing can increase the heart rate and cause dizziness.

■ **Taking blood pressure is an external means of testing how fast the heart is pumping blood around the body.**

■ **Chi Kung relaxes the body, soothes the mind, and therefore calms the heart.**

• BODY IS TOTALLY AT EASE

Fang Sung Kung, or relaxation breathing (*see pp. 72–73*), helps tense muscles to relax and promotes mental tranquility. As such, it is the form of Chi Kung that is best for heart patients. It is usually performed lying down, but if this is difficult for you because of your condition, you can also do it sitting in a chair.

Your breathing rhythm should be as natural and spontaneous as possible.

With each in and out breathing cycle, your body relaxes a bit more. And the effect is cumulative. The relaxation of your body makes your breathing more relaxed. This, in turn, further relaxes your body. With practice, you will be able to achieve a state of deep relaxation and peace. If you perform this exercise 2 or 3 times daily for about 30 minutes each session, you should get good results.

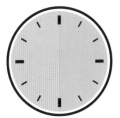

■ Breathing exercises done in half-hour sessions will bring the greatest benefits.

BREATHING IS DONE THROUGH THE NOSE ●

● ALL BODY PARTS ARE RELAXED IN TURN

HANDS REST ● COMFORTABLY ON THE LAP

FEET ARE PARALLEL AND SHOULDER-WIDTH APART ●

■ For heart patients, Fang Sung Kung relaxes the body, which in turn relaxes the breathing.

How Healing Exercise Helps High Blood Pressure

If you practice gentle, regular exercise such as Tai Chi, then the vasodilation caused by the mental and physical relaxation, combined with the rotational movement, will gently invigorate the circulation of the blood, without straining the heart. Over time and with regular practice the heart may regain its health and blood-pressure levels may improve.

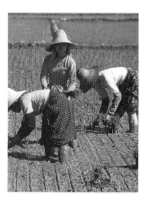

■ **Working in the fields, or any form of manual labor, is good for the heart.**

Statistics show that physically active people, whether athletes or manual laborers, rarely have hypertension, or high blood pressure. And if they do get it, it usually occurs 10 to 15 years later than in those whose jobs require little activity.

But exercise need not be vigorous to help prevent hypertension—people who practice the gentle flowing art of Tai Chi have been shown to have lower blood pressure than their non-exercising counterparts.

Healing exercise fights high blood pressure in a number of ways. The relaxation it produces helps counter overactivity in the cerebral cortex and in the vasomotor center that regulates the size of blood vessels and may cause blood pressure to rise. Physical exercise also lowers sympathetic nerve excitability, which is related to hypertension. And mild exercise, if practiced systematically, can excite the vagus nerve, which slows down the heart.

Therapeutic exercise facilitates blood circulation and improves the body's adaptability. What usually happens is that during exercise, the heart rate and systolic pressure of patients with hypertension rise rapidly. But consistent practice of healing exercise can help moderate these reactions, and the patients can then increase their level of physical activity.

The blood pressure of patients who have mild hypertension generally fluctuates from normal to high. They may typically display symptoms such as headache, dizziness, ringing in the ears, and irritability. However, except for occasional palpitations and shortness of breath, they may not experience any pain around their heart. The most appropriate exercises for them are Tai Chi (*see pp. 60–67*), Chi Kung (*see pp. 68–71*), walking, and self-massage, all of which are mild and slow. They are most beneficial in helping patients achieve their goal of lowering blood pressure, not strengthening the heart. High-intensity exercises may bring about drastic changes in the

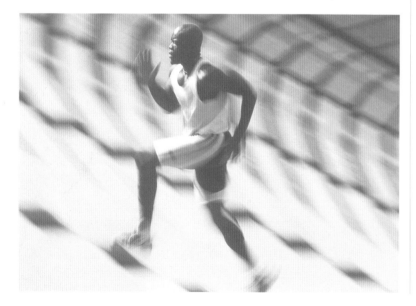

■ **Excessive exercise puts considerable strain on the heart and blood pressure.**

heart rate and blood pressure. Headache and dizziness may also result.

If you have high blood pressure, you should work out a schedule that has a proper balance between activity and inactivity. People with mild hypertension should exercise for about 1 hour a day, 2 or 3 times a week. In each of these sessions, 20 to 30 minutes may be devoted to more demanding exercises. People with moderate high blood pressure should limit their exercise to 30 minutes 2 or 3 days a week. If you wish, you can divide the time into morning and afternoon sessions of 15 minutes each. In between workouts, stay relatively inactive.

Tai Chi and high blood pressure

Tai Chi regulates blood flow, heart function, and activity of the nervous system, all of which are interdependent and influence each other. So regular daily practice of Tai Chi can help to alleviate high blood pressure, as well as calming and soothing the emotions.

■ The body systems are all intricately linked by means of veins, arteries and nerves.

RESPIRATORY CENTER (CONTROLS BREATHING RATE, ETC)

POSITION OF CAROTID SINUS AND CAROTID BODY

RIGHT VAGUS NERVE

ARTERY

LIVER

STOMACH

Cautions for those with high blood pressure

✳ If, in addition to high blood pressure, you have medical complications such as serious arrhythmia, tachycardia, vasospasm, or angina pectoris, then you should not engage in therapeutic exercise unless supervised by a doctor.

✳ You should not participate in exercises that raise the heart rate above 125 beats per minute.

✳ While exercising, you should stay relaxed and avoid tensing your muscles.

✳ Breathe naturally and try not to hold your breath.

✳ Do not do weight-lifting or carry any heavy objects.

✳ Try to keep your head up in order to avoid dizziness.

✳ Symptoms such as chest pain, headache, dizziness, arrhythmia, coughing, and vomiting are all signals to stop the exercise for the time being and consult your doctor.

✳ If the workout is strenuous, you should note your heart rate. Usually your heart rate should return to the normal pre-exercise level about 5 minutes after you have finished the exercise.

✳ Fatigue from exercise will almost always dissipate after 2 hours of rest. If you continue to feel tired, it may mean that the intensity level was too high and you need to make some adjustments.

✳ If you exercise indoors, make sure you do it in an open quiet space.

✳ Be sure to stay in close contact with a health professional and to learn more about both the principles and techniques of physical exercise.

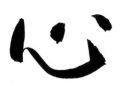

(14)

FANG SONG YUN DONG

Relaxation Exercises

The fundamental goals of Chi Kung are to relax, calm, and recenter energy. This ancient collection of breathing techniques works on hypertension by inhibiting overactivity of the sympathetic nervous system, while activating the parasympathetic system. The sympathetic system responds to stress by speeding up the heart rate, increasing blood pressure, and generally preparing the body for action. The parasympathetic system, by contrast, slows the heart rate, decreases blood pressure, and stimulates the digestive system. A proper balance between these two parts of the autonomic nervous system helps to reduce blood pressure.

There are many Chi Kung techniques. One is a simple relaxation exercise. While sitting in a chair and breathing naturally and spontaneously, silently repeat the words "calm" and "relaxed" to yourself. Picture every part of your body relaxing, from your head to your feet. Feel the tension lessen in your nerves, heart, and blood vessels.

Another easy Chi Kung technique, called three-circle Chi Kung, can be done standing with your feet shoulder-width apart, your knees slightly bent, and your back straight. Hold your arms in front of you as if you were gently holding a globe around its equator. As you breathe deeply, let calming images flow through your mind: you could picture a warm glow of healing energy spreading through your body, or see yourself playing in a beautiful, open space outside, with the sun on your skin. You feel serene and happy.

■ **Visualizing soothing scenes from nature can help in the relaxation process.**

SOOTHING WORDS ARE
REPEATED SILENTLY

BREATHING IS
NATURAL AND
SPONTANEOUS

THE WHOLE BODY IS
GRADUALLY RELAXED

Physically weak patients may alternate standing and sitting breathing exercises. Gradually increase the time given to the standing exercise from about 3 minutes to about 20 minutes. If you become tired, stop and take a rest.

The standing breathing exercise seems to be more effective in the treatment of high blood pressure than the sitting one, perhaps because the standing position better corrects what Chinese doctors call the solid-top-but-empty-bottom syndrome. This syndrome—which is characterized by a sensation of congestion and swelling in the head while the lower regions may feel sore and easily tired, and the feet may be unsteady—is common in patients with hypertension.

The standing exercise stimulates the muscles of the legs and fixes the center of gravity in the lower body. It also helps recenter *chi*, or energy. You can imagine your energy moving down from your head to your abdomen and then to the soles of your feet. This self-suggestion, combined with the muscle contraction and breathing, redirects the blood flow to the lower limbs, reducing congestion in the head and lowering blood pressure. Patients feel fresh and unburdened mentally. Their legs feel stronger and steadier.

To get the best results, hypertensive patients need to practice Chi Kung systematically and regularly so that all parts of the body become less subject to irritation and therefore more relaxed.

AN IMAGINARY GLOBE IS HELD IN THE HANDS

FEET ARE SHOULDER-WIDTH APART

More Exercise to Lower Blood Pressure

If you can help to heal yourself by means of simple lifestyle changes and self-help, such as exercise, you can reduce the need for medication and surgery, and make a positive step toward regaining your mental and physical health. There are various forms of exercise to lower blood pressure, but you must be careful to choose something appropriate for your age and health.

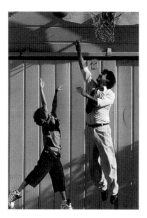

■ **Shooting basketballs into a net can be enjoyable as well as therapeutic.**

Tai Chi, therapeutic gymnastics, leisure walking, and swimming can all help people who have hypertension. Patients who have mild cases may also jog and hike if they do so carefully—set realistic targets and stop immediately if any discomfort is experienced.

✲ **Tai Chi:** Its gentleness and smooth, harmonious movements make Tai Chi an ideal exercise for hypertensive patients. It generates mental concentration and produces peacefulness; it is also totally without force or pressure. Muscle relaxation induced by Tai Chi helps establish a conditioned relaxation reflex in the blood vessels, which lowers blood pressure. Patients who are physically fit may perform the whole set of simplified Tai Chi (*see pp. 62–67*). Weaker patients should do only half of it; those who are very weak or who have a poor memory may simply practice some of the movement exercises (*see pp. 60–61*) without necessarily following the entire sequence.

A good workout routine for patients with high blood pressure might include breathing exercises, relaxation techniques, gentle stretching

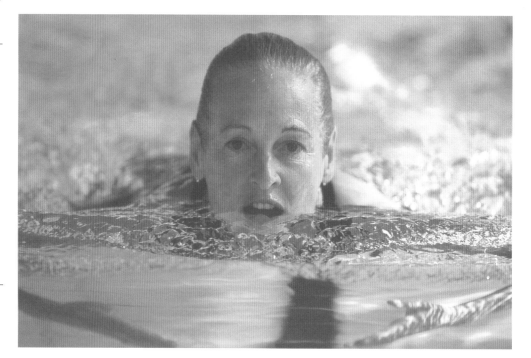

■ **Swimming, being non-weight-bearing, is good for those who are less fit, but it should not be too strenuous.**

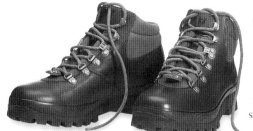

■ **Hiking should be quite gentle and done mainly on the flat or on very slight inclines.**

and reaching exercises for the limbs and torso, walking, and games. A few movements from Tai Chi could be included between exercises. The entire session should last 20 to 30 minutes and should be done once or twice a day, in a group or individually.

✳ **Walking**: Regular walking can help lower systolic blood pressure. It is best to walk at a moderate speed on level ground once or twice a day, for 15 minutes to an hour, depending on your condition. Morning and early evening are both suitable times for walking, as it is generally cooler then.

✳ **Swimming**: Because the weight of the body is supported by the water, swimming is a good exercise for those who are less fit. For maximum benefit, keep your body movements slow and gentle.

✳ **Games**: Choose sports that are relaxing and fun, such as shooting basketballs or badminton. If you are by nature extremely competitive and feel cross with yourself every time you miss a shot, you may be better doing swimming or walking instead.

✳ **Jogging and fast walking**: The intensity level of these exercises is relatively high, causing a hypertensive patient's pulse rate to rise significantly. Therefore, use caution in deciding if such exercise is suitable for you. It may be best to start by walking for ½–1 mile (1–2km) at a speed of 16 to 20 minutes per mile (8 to 10 minutes per km). If there are no ill effects, you may intensify your walking or try gentle jogging. Remember that

■ **Tai Chi is the ideal exercise for those with hypertension—from those who are weak to the physically fit.**

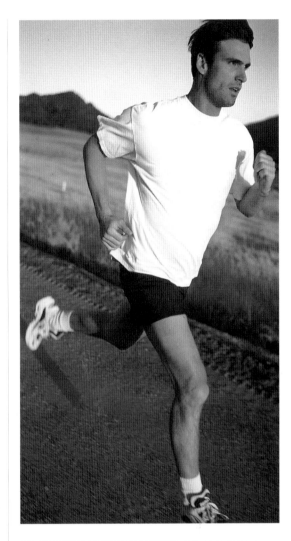

■ **Jogging is a high-impact activity and should be carefully monitored.**

you should monitor your heart rate. It is normal for it to increase by 20 to 30 beats per minute immediately after exercise.

✳ **Hiking**: If high blood pressure is not complicated by other problems, then young people whose condition is mild may do some gentle hiking, with plenty of walking on the flat interspersed between mild gradients. Start by attempting an incline of 30 or 45 degrees for a distance of no more than 50yd (50m). Follow this exertion with a rest period if fatigue results. Do not attempt to do too much too quickly.

Exercise and Hardening of the Arteries

The composition of the wall of the arteries is affected by the composition of the blood and, as blood is nourished by the food that we eat, attention to correct diet will ensure good health. For the health of the blood, arteries and heart we should be eating far more fruit and vegetables than we generally do, as well as practicing Tai Chi and other forms of exercise.

The coronary artery is one of the most important blood vessels in the body because it supplies blood to the heart. If this artery, or any others, begins to harden, it loses its elasticity and blood flow around the body is impeded. Proper exercise can both help prevent and treat hardening of the arteries, also known as arteriosclerosis. According to several studies, physically active people are less likely to have hardening of the arteries and are less likely to develop coronary disease than people who don't exercise.

Exercise helps in at least two ways. The relief it provides from mental tension can minimize the risk of vasospasm, a condition in which vessels cramp and shut, preventing blood flow. And exercise is closely related to the level of cholesterol in the blood—it is a significant factor in lowering the level of artery-clogging cholesterol.

The healing exercises recommended for patients with arteriosclerosis are basically the same as those for patients with high blood pressure, many of whom also have arteriosclerosis. If, however, the arteriosclerosis is severe, exercise should be lighter and the method and style simpler than that for hypertensives. Good exercises are walking for pleasure, simplified Tai Chi, therapeutic gymnastics, and massage. The total time that is devoted to exercise should not exceed 45 minutes per day.

❈ **Walking:** The best time for walking in the summer is in the morning or evening, to avoid the midday heat. Walk in a peaceful environment, if possible for ¼–½ mile (400–800m). Aim to complete this sort of distance in 5 to 10 minutes. This kind of slow walking will help you sleep well and improve your digestion.

❈ **Tai Chi:** Depending on your physical condition, you can either practice the entire set (*see pp. 62–67*), do a half set, or just do some of the individual movements.

■ **Massage performed by a professional can aid circulation to the limbs.**

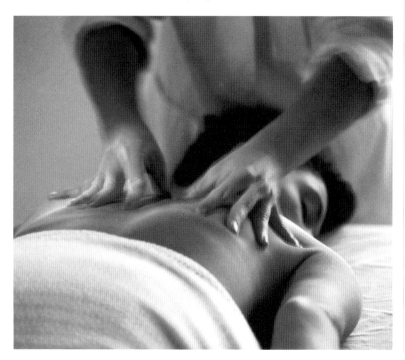

Hardening of the arteries

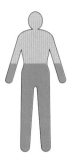

■ It is possible to lower cholesterol levels in the blood after exercising each day for a minimum of 2 months.

Hardening of the arteries occurs when a build-up of what is known as "atheromatous plaque"—comprising fats circulating in the blood, and particularly cholesterol—occurs on the wall of the artery. This impedes the flow of blood through the artery and, when it becomes large enough, can cause the blood to dam up behind it, resulting in a blood clot or thrombosis. By avoiding excessive amounts of fatty food and eating more fruit and vegetables, we can improve the quality of our blood composition and thereby reduce the risk of arteriosclerosis.

■ A clot occurs when a build-up of fatty deposits starts to block the artery and prevent blood from flowing freely.

NORMAL ARTERY

BUILD-UP OF ATHEROMATOUS PLAQUE

FATTY CORE

FURTHER BUILD-UP CAUSING TURBULENCE AND CLOT FORMATION

CORONARY ARTERY

CORONARY ARTERY

■ The coronary arteries bring blood to the muscle cells of the heart, providing them with fuel and oxygen.

15

ZHI LIAO YING TI CAO JI AN MA

Therapeutic Gymnastics and Massage

The goal in therapeutic gymnastics and massage is to improve your physical condition generally, especially blood circulation in the limbs. For all of the exercises that follow, sit on a chair with your feet on the floor and your back straight. A straight spine is essential to good Chi Kung.

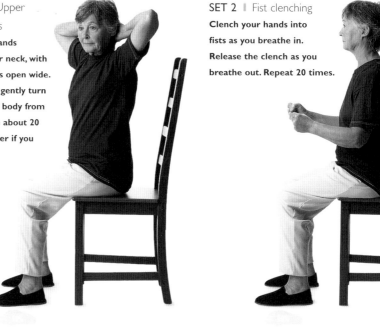

SET 1 | Upper body turns
Put both hands behind your neck, with your elbows open wide. Slowly and gently turn your upper body from side to side about 20 times—fewer if you feel dizzy.

SET 2 | Fist clenching
Clench your hands into fists as you breathe in. Release the clench as you breathe out. Repeat 20 times.

ESSENTIAL POINTS

■ Stretch only as far as is comfortable—do not overexert yourself.

■ The moves will flex different parts of the body; try and keep as relaxed as possible.

SET 3 | Foot circling
Lift your feet from the floor and stretch your legs out in front of you. Hold onto the edge of the chair and make tiny circles with your feet, first clockwise, then counterclockwise. Be sure not to overtire yourself.

SET 4 | Leg extensions
Hold onto the edge of the seat at the front. Extend each leg, in turn, straight out in front of you. Hold it there for a few seconds.

SET 5 ▮ Waist bending

Stretch both legs in front of you, keeping your heels on the floor. Put your hands on your thighs. Then bend at the waist and slide your hands down your legs as you breathe out. Breathe in as you straighten up and draw your hands back. Repeat several times.

SET 6 ▮ Self-massage

Massage should be done early in the morning or at bedtime; it can also be done after exercise. Massage your head region first, rubbing your fingertips into your scalp in small circular movements. Then form your right hand into a loose fist and beat your left shoulder for a few moments, before moving on down the arm. Do the same with your left hand and right shoulder. Then clap your palms moderately hard on your thighs for several minutes. Bending at the waist, clap your open palms down the legs from top to bottom, all the way down to the feet.

RIGHT FIST BEATS
THE LEFT ARM

1

2

Coronary Artery Disease and Healing Exercise

Reports from China and other countries indicate that people over the age of 40 who exercise frequently are far less likely to have coronary artery disease—an increasingly common problem—than those who are inactive; and even when they do suffer, healing exercise gives them a much greater chance of recovery than their chair-bound contemporaries.

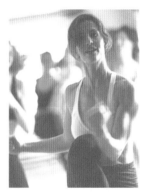

■ **Aerobic exercise increases the intake of oxygen, which is beneficial for those with coronary artery disease.**

Coronary artery disease is characterized by a thickening of the walls of the vessels that supply the heart, reducing the flow of blood. Because of inadequate blood supply, the heart muscle does not get enough oxygen. The patient may feel a squeezing or pressing pain in the center of the chest, which may radiate to the arm, neck, or jaw and be accompanied by shortness of breath. If the obstruction takes place suddenly, and there is prolonged shortage of blood to the heart muscle, myocardial infarction—heart attack—results.

Physical inactivity and the onset of coronary artery disease appear to be related. In recent years, therapeutic exercises for coronary disease have been developed and used in many parts of the world with beneficial results. For patients who have not suffered heart attacks, exercise therapy can help improve fitness and speed up recovery from clogged arteries.

Exercise facilitates oxygen supply to the heart muscle by promoting and improving collateral circulation. It actually reduces the heart's demand for oxygen by increasing the organ's efficiency. It improves lipometabolism, or the body's use of

■ **Gentle movements, such as Drawing a Bow (see p.49), are therapeutic and relaxing.**

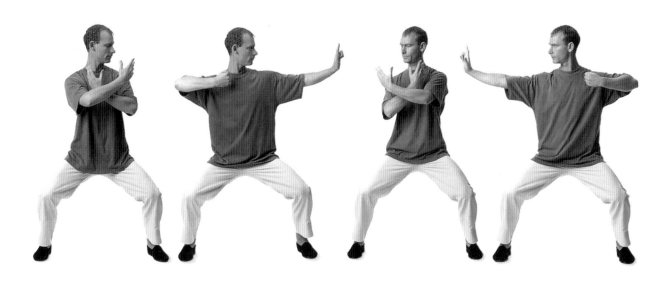

fats. Regular systematic exercise helps lower the serum cholesterol level and reduces cholesterol build-up on the artery walls. It also helps break up clots of fibrin—a natural protein substance—into soluble fragments in the blood. This reduces the likelihood of clotting in the vessels. Above all, exercise improves attitude. Not only does it direct attention away from disease but it also gives a sense of health, control, and optimism. All of these help prevent the recurrence of painful angina pectoris and other heart problems.

A key factor in treating coronary disease with exercise is to determine the optimal amount and type of exercise. If the level of intensity is too low, then the exercise will not improve heart efficiency. If it is too high, it may trigger angina or other symptoms—or, in fact, even endanger life. Always consult your doctor about a suitable program before starting exercise.

Heart rate may be the best guide for determining the optimal level of exercise intensity. Heart rate, oxygen absorption, and the capacity

■ An electrocardiogram measures the electrical activity of the heart.

for physical exertion are all related. And the heart rate seems to be the most accurate indicator of how much oxygen is absorbed by the heart muscle, as well as how much blood is circulating through the coronary artery. So, to determine the optimal level of intensity at which to exercise, you should determine your maximum heart rate—that is, your heart rate during maximum physical exertion—and multiply this by 80 percent. Maximum heart rate is normally calculated by subtracting your age from 200. Look at the charts to help you discover your desired heart rate during exercise and suitable exercises to achieve this.

Heart rates for coronary patients during healing exercise

AGE	MAXIMUM HEART RATE (MHR) DURING EXERCISE (200 MINUS AGE)	IDEAL HEART RATE DURING EXERCISE (80% OF MHR)
35	165	132
40	160	128
45	155	124
50	150	120
55	145	116
60	140	112
65	135	108
70	130	104

Typical heart rates for different exercises

EXERCISE	HEART RATE
Simplified Tai Chi	90 to 105
Fast walking	100 to 110
Swimming 100yd (100m) at medium speed	105 to 108
Table tennis	95 to 126
Jogging (medium distance)	120 to 140
Soccer, basketball	140 to 180
Martial arts	150 to 172
Running (medium/long distance)	180

Exercises for Coronary Artery Disease

If we can keep chi flowing smoothly, this will keep the blood flowing smoothly. To gently mobilize chi we can do Tai Chi (sometimes called "swimming in the air") or Chi Kung; to mobilize it more forcefully we can do fast walking or swimming. When the body flows in a smooth, continuous way on the outside, blood and chi will be flowing smoothly on the inside.

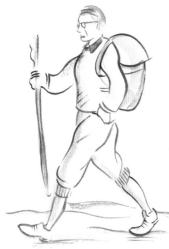

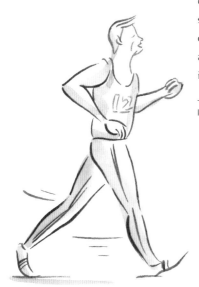

■ Walk fast for about 45 minutes per day.

Depending on your age, your physical condition and personal preferences, you can choose one or more of the following exercises to help improve your health and act as a preventative to further arterial damage.

❋ **Walking:** Fast walking—100 steps per minute—has a greater impact on the heart than leisurely walking. It can raise the pulse to 100 beats a minute or even higher. You should choose a pace and a step length that feel comfortable and let you breathe naturally. Don't be afraid to slow down if you find you are getting tired—you will still be getting the benefits. If walking is your only exercise, gradually try to aim for a total time of at least 45 minutes a day, broken into two sessions if you wish.

■ Swim for up to 40 minutes, 2 or 3 times a week.

❋ **Slow jogging:** Slow jogging is appropriate for people who are fit—that is, who have regularly done other types of exercises. You can jog a short distance—50–200yd (50–200m)—or a long distance—up to 2 miles (3.2km). Monitor your heart rate and keep it under 120 beats per minute. Of course, if angina pain occurs following long-distance jogging, choose another exercise.

❋ **Pace-determined walking:** The first section of this exercise is better for people whose disease is more severe. As you gain strength, you can keep adding portions, until you are doing the whole course.

Start by walking on level ground for 3000yd (3000m). Complete the first third in 20 minutes and then rest for 5 minutes. Do the next third in 16 to 18 minutes followed by a 5-minute rest. Allow yourself 20 minutes for the final third.

■ Do pace-determined walking, timing yourself as you go.

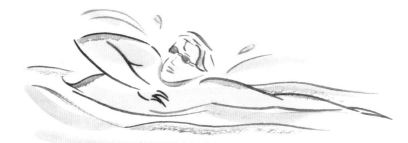

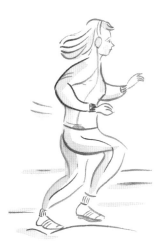

■ **Jog slowly, aiming to keep your heart rate under 120 beats per minute.**

Next walk on level ground for 4000yd (4000m). Complete half the distance in about 40 minutes, including a 5-minute break at the halfway point. Then walk on a hill with a 30-degree to 45-degree slope for about 30 minutes. Take a break for 5 to 10 minutes, then walk down the slope, and back the way you came, as before.

❋ **Swimming:** If you have moderate physical strength and enjoy swimming, this could be the ideal exercise for you, as it seems to improve the body's ability to absorb oxygen. The typical heart rates are the same as those for fast walking, but there is no jarring of the joints, as swimming is non-weight-bearing. Aim to swim for about 20 minutes 2 or 3 times a week and build this up gradually to 30 or 40 minutes per session.

❋ **Chi Kung:** Practice Fang Sung Kung, relaxation breathing (*see pp. 72–73*), or Chiang Chuang Kung, invigorating breathing (*see pp. 74–77*), either sitting or lying down. Don't try to breathe too deeply or to hold your breath. Chi Kung is especially helpful for patients who are weak and nervous. You can expect this exercise to improve the circulation in your extremities and produce warmth in the limbs. You may also get relief from dizziness, improve your mood, and decrease the frequency and intensity of any anginal pain.

❋ **Tai Chi:** Composed of soft movements and easy relaxed postures, Tai Chi (*see pp. 60–67*) is excellent for heart patients who have high blood pressure. It also calms the nerves.

■ **Rest for 10 minutes or longer after exercising.**

Precautions for coronary patients doing healing exercise

✱ Coronary patients who have angina pectoris and those recovering from heart attacks should consult their doctor about the amount and type of exercise that they may do.

✱ Always do warm-up exercises before and cool-down exercises after each training session. Engaging in high-intensity exercises without warming up may trigger angina. Stopping the exercise abruptly without first relaxing and letting your heart rate slow gradually may also cause discomfort in the heart region.

✱ Never overstretch yourself to pursue a so-called maximum or optimal heart rate.

✱ Before each exercise session take your pulse by counting for 10 seconds and multiplying by 6. Measure it again when you are exercising most vigorously and once more 2 minutes after you stop exercising. Use this information to monitor your body and to adjust the level of intensity of the exercise.

✱ If you experience shortness of breath or dizziness during exercise, take longer breaks between intervals or perform rhythmic breathing exercises every now and then.

✱ If you feel extremely fatigued and experience chest congestion, shortness of breath, internal pressure or pain in the region of the heart, the upper left arm, or the left side of the neck, then you should stop exercising immediately and consult your doctor.

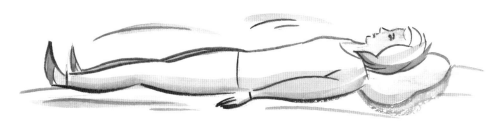

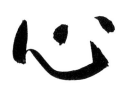

16

BA GE SHI BING

Buerger's Disease

Thromboangitis obliterans, also known as Buerger's disease, is a circulatory disorder that affects the smaller arteries and veins, and is marked by inflammation, deterioration of the blood vessels, and clotting. The disease prevents the tissues from getting an adequate supply of blood, oxygen, and nutrients, and, in the most severe cases, gangrene may develop. The causes of Buerger's disease are not fully known, but it is definitely associated with smoking. Traditional Chinese doctors attribute the condition to *chi* deficiency, blood and *chi* stagnation, and inadequate nourishment, with too many heavily seasoned and greasy foods. The early symptoms of Buerger's disease, which occurs chiefly in young men, are feelings of cold and numbness in the extremities. The patient's legs turn pale and feel heavy and weak, and he may limp. At night the sufferer feels extreme pain. During the late stages of this disease, the patient can no longer feel anything in the affected limb because of tissue deterioration.

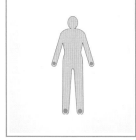

ESSENTIAL POINTS

- Gently invigorate the circulation.
- Make sure that you also pay attention to eating the correct diet

LEGS ARE AT 45 DEGREES TO THE BED

SET 1 | Foot stretching

Lie on your back on your bed and raise your legs to form a 45-degree angle. Hold this position for 1 to 2 minutes.

2 **Then dangle your legs over the edge of the bed for 2 to 5 minutes. Stretch your toes and move your feet at the same time. Rotate your ankles up and down, pointing the feet in and out, at least 10 times.**

ANKLES ARE ROTATED UP AND DOWN

Because healing exercise strengthens muscles and blood vessels and facilitates circulation, it can help non-smokers prevent this disease. And in the early stages, therapeutic exercise can help control the affliction, especially when used in conjunction with other therapies such as acupuncture and Chinese herbal medicine.

If the legs are affected, the best exercises are walking on level ground for 30 minutes daily, stretching, callisthenics, Tai Chi, or canoeing.

SET 2 | Arm and leg shaking

Lie on your back and lift your arms and legs straight into the air. Gently shake your limbs in this position for 1 to 2 minutes. Lower your limbs and rest, then repeat 5 or 6 times. This should be repeated at intervals 3 to 5 times a day.

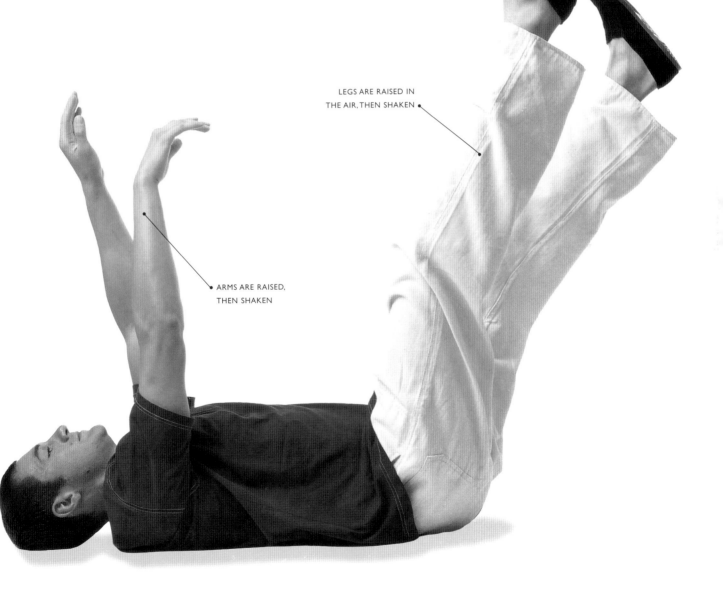

LEGS ARE RAISED IN THE AIR, THEN SHAKEN

ARMS ARE RAISED, THEN SHAKEN

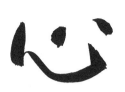

(17)

SHI BING DONG SHOU JU HE NUAN

Warming Cold Hands and Cold Feet

In summer as well as winter, some people suffer from ice-cold hands and feet. The condition may be caused by physical weakness and inadequate blood circulation in the capillaries. But in most cases, the body's temperature regulation system is not working properly.

In summer, people with this syndrome perspire so much that their hands and feet are constantly moist and chilly. In winter, their bodies—trying to conserve energy and keep them warm—constrict the smaller arteries and reduce the flow of blood to peripheral areas.

This syndrome can be helped through various types of healing exercises. Massage can improve peripheral blood circulation in the limbs. Either pound your arms and legs with a loose fist or clap them repeatedly with an open palm.

To correct the underlying cause, however, you need to improve your overall physical strength, together with your body temperature-regulating mechanism. This can only be done through the systematic and persistent practice of a vigorous exercise program, such as fast walking or cycling.

Chi Kung (*see pp. 68–71*) and Tai Chi (*see pp. 60–67*) can also be used to treat this condition. According to one study, skin temperatures of both hands and feet—measured both objectively and by the feelings of the patients themselves—were higher during Chi Kung and Tai Chi practice.

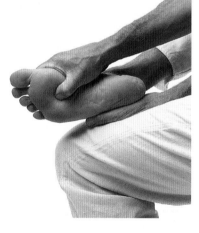

ESSENTIAL POINTS

■ Eat sufficient hot food in winter to supply the body with energy for warmth.

■ 70 percent of body heat is lost through the head, so wear a hat if you are exercising outdoors.

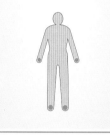

To improve circulation in the limbs, clap the arms and legs repeatedly with an open palm. This should be accompanied by a calm but concentrated state of mind.

Coldness in the feet can be counteracted by rubbing the acupuncture point known as Yung Chuan (Bubbling Spring), which is located one-third of the way down the foot, in the depression formed when the toes are curled under (see pp. 58–59). Do this immediately after getting up in the morning and just before going to bed. Continue rubbing until the foot becomes warm.

HOW PURPURA CAN BE PREVENTED WITH HEALING EXERCISE

Purpura is a bleeding disease in which blood leeches into the skin, the subcutaneous tissues, and the mucous membranes. It causes bruiselike purplish or reddish blotches. Unfortunately, thrombocytopenic purpura and allergic purpura—two common forms of the disease—cannot be treated by therapeutic exercise. In fact, serious cases call for bed rest.

Thrombocytopenic purpura can be identified by a deficiency in blood platelets and a prolonged clotting time. The blood platelet count often falls below 50,000 per cc. of blood. Allergic purpura, which frequently has a sudden onset, usually shows a normal platelet count and normal coagulation. Purplish spots may appear on the skin of the lower extremities as well as pale or red wheals. Severe abdominal pain, swollen and painful joints, and blood with the stool or urine are also seen in cases of severe allergic purpura.

But the third type of purpura can be helped by exercise. It is a type that is frequently overlooked or misdiagnosed. Caused by blockage of blood in the veins—the result of prolonged sitting or standing—Chinese doctors describe it as being characterized by swollen and painful dark purple patches on the legs. Platelet count and coagulation time appear to be normal.

Physical exercises such as callisthenics and stretching, walking, Tai Chi, and therapeutic gymnastics for the legs prevent this type of purpura—and they can even cure it. The symptoms usually disappear a week or so after you begin exercising.

SET 1 | Upper body twists

Place both your hands behind your neck, with your elbows pushed backward. Slowly twist your upper body from side to side. Do this about 20 times—but fewer if it makes you feel dizzy.

SET 2 | Making fists

Breathe in and clench your hands into fists as you do so, then relax the hands as you breathe out. Repeat 20 times.

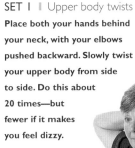

CHAPTER FOUR

Combating lung and respiratory disease through healing exercise

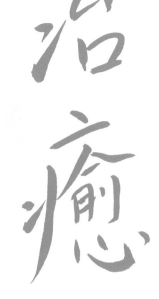

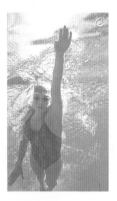

Swimming can considerably increase our ability to absorb oxygen.

The respiratory system is a sophisticated mechanism but, like all such body systems, is delicate and subject to disorders, ranging from simple coughs and colds to bronchitis, emphysema, and asthma. Asthma in particular has been on the increase in recent years, while many of the complaints that afflict the respiratory system are self-inflicted, largely through smoking (whether voluntary or passive). However, doctors in China have proven that exercise can benefit people with lung problems.

In traditional Chinese medicine the lungs are considered to govern the inhalation and exhalation of *chi*, and not just oxygen, and as we have already seen, when *chi* is flowing smoothly and is in harmony, the body will be healthy. The lungs are also seen as being responsible for dispersing body fluids to the kidneys, so impaired lung function may result in fluid retention and swelling in parts of the body. But help is at hand for those suffering from respiratory complaints, in the form of healing exercise, massage, and breathing exercises.

Even those with asthma and bronchitis can be helped by healing exercise.

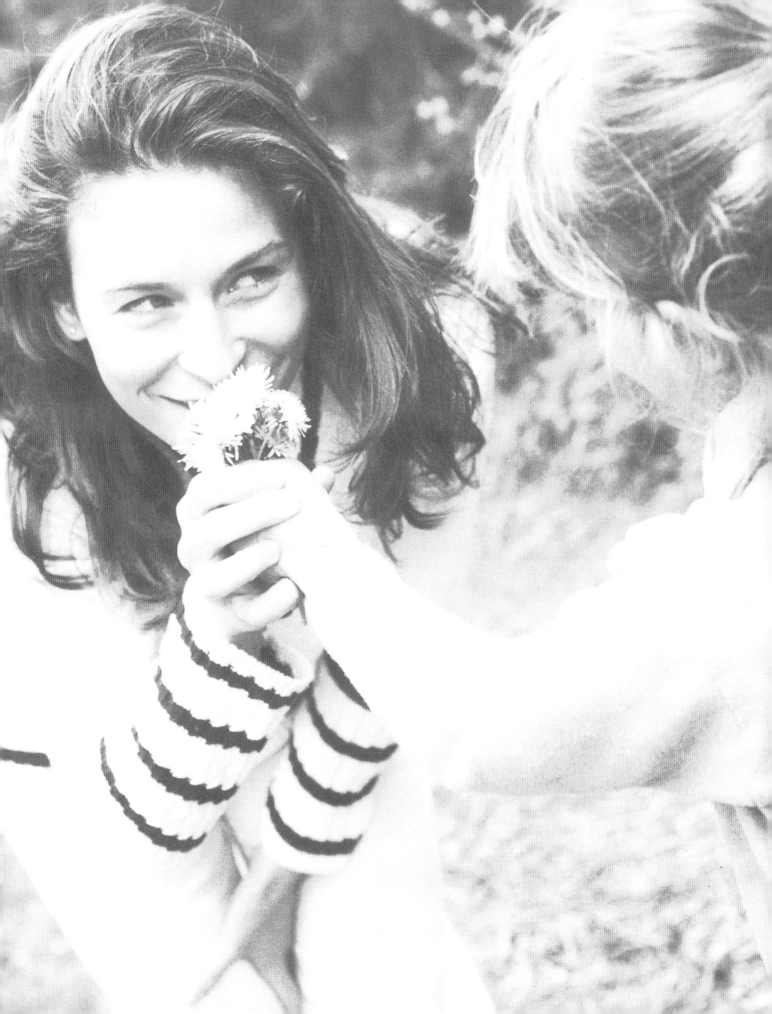

Breathe Easier with Healing Exercise

Chi Kung (also known as The Art of Breathing) is extremely beneficial in healing respiratory problems, especially when it is combined with Tai Chi. Breathing correctly assists in the oxygenation of the blood and increases the amount of chi *in the body. But we must exercise the whole body to strengthen respiration, for breathing is not just to do with the lungs.*

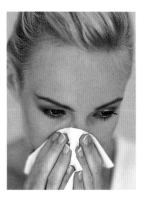

■ **Coughs and colds are one of the most common manifestations of respiratory problems.**

Doctors and physical fitness experts believe that both deep breathing exercises and other activities can benefit people with lung problems—even some of the most serious ones.

One measure of lung health is vital capacity—the maximum volume of air that can be exhaled after a full inhalation. For adult women, this amount is usually in the range of 2500–3000ml; for men, it is 3500–4000ml. If vital capacity is too low—below 2000–2500ml—which is often the case in those with lung diseases such as pneumonia, emphysema, or bronchitis, these people may feel shortness of breath during exercise or physical labor.

Deep breathing exercises can increase vital capacity, but they may not significantly improve respiration overall. The most effective exercises for stimulating lung function, according to studies done in physical education, include swimming, canoeing, basketball, and jogging—exercises that demand the greatest performance from the whole respiratory system. A basketball player, for example, breathes 7 to 14 times the volume of air

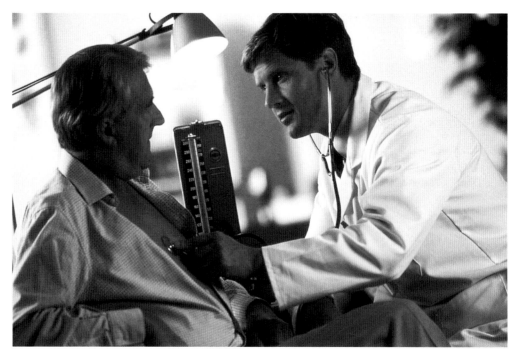

■ **Examination by stethoscope can reveal much about the condition of the lungs.**

used while resting, and a runner takes in 15 to 20 times more air than during a rest period.

Other factors also play a role. Swimming and canoeing can help develop the chest muscles, for instance. And water pressure against the chest while you are swimming is believed to strengthen respiratory ability.

Lung and circulatory problems frequently occur together and make vigorous exercise too risky for those who are suffering from both complaints. But Tai Chi, walking, and slow jogging—simple, easy exercises that can be practiced all year-round— can be extremely helpful even to those who are not able to do vigorous exercise.

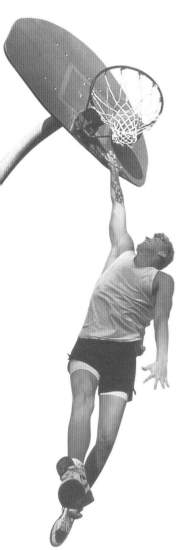

■ **Basketball exercises the whole respiratory system and is highly beneficial.**

CAUTION
People who have breathing or lung problems should not take part in strenuous activities without consulting their doctor.

Preventing the common cold with self-massage

More than a thousand years ago, the Chinese discovered that cold-induced nasal congestion could be relieved by massaging both sides of the bridge of the nose. Later, acupuncturists learned that nasal congestion could also be eased by stimulating the Yin Shen (Welcome Fragrance) point on each side of the nose. These findings led to the discovery that colds could in fact be prevented simply by massaging these points systematically. It is thought that massage probably improves blood circulation and metabolism in the mucous membranes, increasing resistance to bacterial invasion.

✱ Rub both sides of the bridge of the nose with your index fingers until the spot feels quite warm.

✱ Rub the Feng Chih (Windy Lake) point on each side of the neck with your palms 30 to 60 times.

■ **Points on either side of the nose may be stimulated to relieve congestion.**

✱ Press on the Yin Shen points on each side of the nose, near the most prominent part of the nostrils. Lightly rub this area with the tip of your index finger for 1 to 3 minutes.

✱ Rub the chest. Using the nipple as the center of a circle, massage the left breast with the right palm and vice versa. Make 10 to 20 circles on each side.

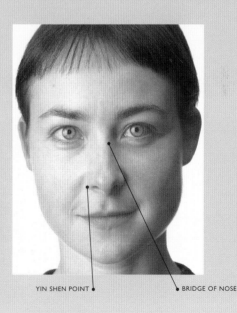

YIN SHEN POINT ●

● BRIDGE OF NOSE

FENG CHIH
(WINDY LAKE)
POINT

■ **The back of the neck can be massaged to bring relief from colds.**

Chronic Obstructive Pulmonary Disease

When combined with Chi Kung, Tai Chi has been shown to aid in the recovery from chronic obstructive pulmonary disease. Taking care to avoid extreme weather conditions of any kind is also important, because hot, dry air will make a dry cough worse, while cold, damp weather will exacerbate phlegm in the chest.

Chronic obstructive pulmonary disease refers to a family of lung disorders that gradually result in a decrease in lung function and increased difficulty in breathing. The most common forms are emphysema and chronic bronchitis, both of which are frequently accompanied by asthma.

Emphysema is characterized by a gradual destruction of the small air sacs, or alveoli, in the lungs. In the alveoli, oxygen passes into the bloodstream for circulation around the body and waste carbon dioxide leaves the blood to be discharged in exhaled air. As these small air sacs degenerate, the surface area over which oxygen and carbon dioxide exchange occurs shrinks. The tissues become weak and less elastic. This leads to a breakdown in the lung structure, which makes exhaling increasingly difficult. When inflated unevenly with air, the lungs display constricted pulmonary emphysema. The classic symptom of this disease is breathlessness.

Chronic bronchitis is a condition in which the air passages in the lungs—the bronchi—become inflamed. The inflammation results in mucus production in the bronchi and smaller tubes—the bronchioles—which become clogged and narrower and smaller, making it difficult for air to pass through. The patient then experiences difficulty in inhaling and exhaling. A chronic bronchitis patient usually has a nagging cough, thick mucus, and may also be breathless.

The term "asthma" refers to a reversible narrowing or spasm of the bronchial airways. This may be caused by allergic reactions, by stress, infection, or simply by the inflammation that is already present in chronic bronchitis patients. Asthma frequently causes wheezing, coughing, and mucus production.

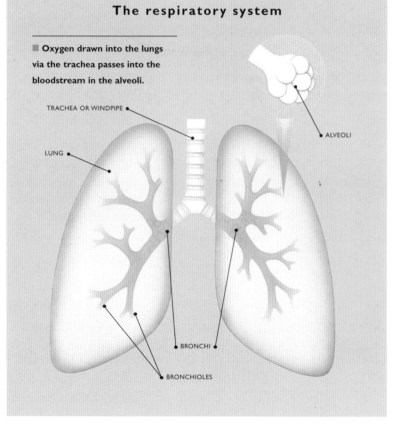

The respiratory system

■ Oxygen drawn into the lungs via the trachea passes into the bloodstream in the alveoli.

TRACHEA OR WINDPIPE

ALVEOLI

LUNG

BRONCHI

BRONCHIOLES

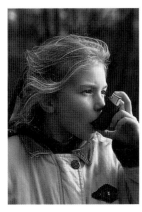

■ **Asthma among the young is increasingly common, often requiring the use of inhalers.**

Deterioration of the ability to breathe may be complicated by infectious diseases involving the respiratory tract, such as pneumonia. Over a period of time, the heart function can also be adversely affected and eventually heart disease may follow. However, along with traditional medical treatment, many people with respiratory disease can help alleviate their symptoms and prevent their condition from worsening through healing exercise.

Treatment of emphysema should focus on preventing and controlling infection (mainly bronchitis and acute pneumonia), reducing inflammation, alleviating bronchiospasm, improving pulmonary function, and enhancing the patient's overall health. Healing exercise does all these things. Exercises should be chosen by determining the overall level of health of the

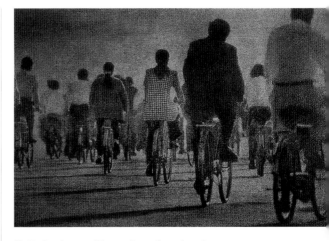

■ **Cycling is a good form of exercise unless the atmosphere is highly polluted.**

individual. Acupuncture and traditional Chinese medicine are both effective in the treatment of respiratory conditions.

Categories of patients with pulmonary emphysema

There are four categories of patients with pulmonary emphysema, classified according to walking ability:

GROUP A
Patients who can walk on level ground as fast as the healthy of the same age and who can body-build. They do not experience shortness of breath when they walk. However, they do not perform as well as their healthy contemporaries when they are walking up and down stairs or over hills.

GROUP B
These patients can walk unhurriedly for ½ mile (1km) without feeling breathless. But they cannot walk as fast as a healthy person on level ground. The best time to begin a therapeutic program is now, when the disease is still in its early stages. Patients can not only get better results now than if the disease was advanced, but they can also prevent it from worsening.

GROUP C
This group of patients will experience shortness of breath after walking on a flat surface for just a few minutes.

GROUP D
These patients—the sickest—feel breathless even when doing simple tasks such as putting on clothes or talking to others.

Patients in groups C and D may benefit from exercise if they proceed in a cautious and systematic manner—and with their doctor's approval—and as long as the disease is not complicated either by acute infection or by serious heart problems.

■ **The ability to walk without getting breathless determines the severity of pulmonary disease.**

Exercises for Those with Emphysema

If a patient does not have access to acupuncture or Chinese herbal medicine, then Tai Chi done in conjunction with Chi Kung will help to alleviate their emphysema. Other healing exercises, such as different forms of massage, can also be helpful in dispelling phlegm, assisting breathing, and relaxing the chest muscles. There is now no doubt that emphysema patients can help themselves.

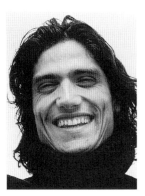

■ **Self-help can improve the life of those with emphysema.**

The best way of treating pulmonary emphysema with exercise emphasizes the body as a whole, rather than merely focusing on improving the lungs. In other words, patients should not restrict themselves to breathing exercises alone, but should also do exercises that benefit the cardiovascular system and overall health. Improving the function of the other organs and the body as a whole will provide the most relief from emphysema symptoms.

Therapeutic exercise for pulmonary emphysema can be divided into three categories:

● Massage, which is used especially to prevent common colds and lessen uncomfortable feelings in the chest.

● Physical fitness exercises to develop endurance, increase strength, and improve general health.

● Breathing exercises that stress the importance of effective respiration, correct bad habits, and encourage muscle relaxation in breathing.

■ **Tai Chi exercises, Chi Kung, and massage make an effective combination.**

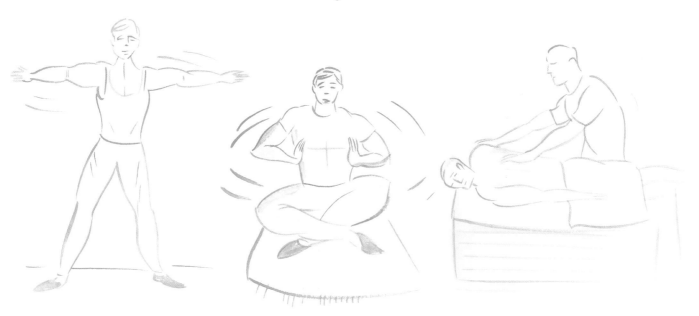

MASSAGING THE CHEST

To achieve the best results, chest massage is usually performed before breathing exercises. Often it can be performed by the patient. But if symptoms are pronounced and the patient is weak, the massage should be done by a medical professional. All of the following methods aid breathing, relax the muscles of the chest wall, and help get rid of phlegm. Massage may be done 2, 3, or more times a day.

SET 2 ▌ Chest clapping

With your right hand shaped as if you were going to applaud, clap the left side of your chest. Work down the outside, across the lower chest, up the front, and finish under the collar bone. Repeat the sequence 3 to 5 times, then clap the right side of your chest with your left hand. If a professional performs this massage, both sides can be done simultaneously.

SET 1 ▌ Vibration massage

Sit in a straight-backed chair and wrap your arms around your chest as if you were hugging yourself. Your hands should be 1–2in (2.5–5cm) below your arms. Now, creating a vibrationlike effect, rub your hands up and down your sides. The motion should be light and swift but with some force. Continue this massage for several minutes.

SET 3 ▌

Rubbing massage

Perform this massage with an open palm, rubbing lightly in a circular motion around the nipple. Use your right hand for your left breast and vice versa. Rubbing as you go, complete 10 to 12 circles.

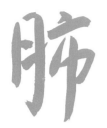

Physical Fitness Exercises for Emphysema Patients

Exercise for those with emphysema should be aimed at building up stamina and strength, and improving general health, because when the overall health of the body is improved, so are the lungs. Invigorating the circulation of the blood and chi through exercise is also essential, so the exercises that follow concentrate on these vital aspects.

❊ **Walking**: Start off by walking ¼–¾ mile (400–1200m) daily, at a pace that is comfortable for you. Divide the distance into three sections: for the first walk slowly; for the middle section increase the speed slightly; and for the final section walk very slowly.

❊ **Walking up and down stairs**: Do this exercise once a day, on steps that are 6–8in (15–20cm) high. On the first day, take 1 step up and 1 step down; on the second day, 2 steps up and 2 steps down. Each succeeding day add another step until 24 steps up and 24 steps down have been reached. Once you have accomplished this goal, gradually reduce the amount of time until you can walk up and down the 24 steps in 18 to 20 seconds.

Patients who are relatively weak can start with the least demanding schedule. Patients who are in better shape may walk up and down stairs for 5 minutes each day.

■ **Walking up and down stairs, in increasing stages, gives you a goal to aim for and achieve.**

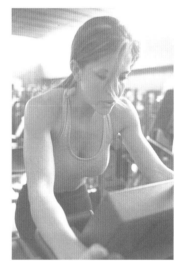

■ **Using an exercise bicycle can slowly build up your strength.**

❊ **Cycling**: Riding an exercise bicycle can help to develop physical endurance. Use a bike with a tension-adjusting device, and to begin with, keep the tension at the lowest setting. The speed should be slow enough not to cause a strain. Practice riding the bicycle for 5 to 7 minutes each day. After a while, you can ride 2 to 3 times daily. Later, practice periods can be increased to 15 to 20 minutes a day, using the same degree of tension. Then gradually increase the tension level. This type of gradual training is extremely beneficial in developing both endurance and stamina.

❊ **Walking at intermittent speeds**: Build strength by varying your walking pace. Walk fast for 30 seconds, followed by a 60-second period of very slow restful walking. Repeat 30 times. This exercise should be done 2 or 3 times a week. After 3 to 6 months you should notice an increase in your physical strength.

Other exercises

Callisthenics and stretching exercises are appropriate for patients who have adequate strength, and Tai Chi (*see pp. 60–67*) can be done by everyone. This relaxing exercise is excellent for relieving feelings of tension and anxiety, which can be induced if you are experiencing difficulty in getting your breath. For developing better lung function, basketball, swimming, hiking, and jogging are great for new patients who are young and otherwise healthy.

■ **Tai Chi is gentle enough not to overstrain the lungs.**

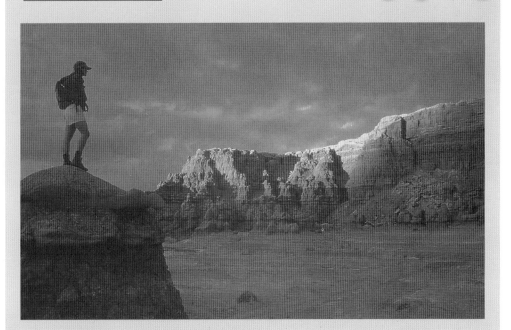

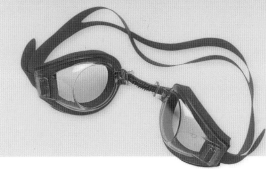

■ **Hiking is a valuable form of exercise and gets you out into the countryside.**

■ **Swimming involves breathing control and will help to regulate the lungs.**

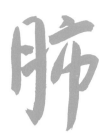

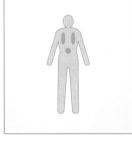

ESSENTIAL POINTS

- For total relaxation let your breath move the belly, rather than your muscles.
- Do not hold yourself up—let the ground support you.

18

HU XI YUN DONG

Breathing Exercises

Emphysema patients can benefit in a number of ways from breathing exercises. The exercises strengthen the muscles involved in breathing, especially the diaphragm. Having lost some of its flexibility while under chronic stress, the diaphragm needs help to regain its mobility. Only a small improvement in the diaphragm can mean a big gain in breathing. If the diaphragm's expandability increases by ⅜in (1cm), studies show, lung capacity grows by 250ml. A ¾in (2cm) increase in the diaphragm can be achieved over time, with the corresponding exponential growth in lung capacity.

These exercises also help develop the habit of abdominal breathing, a method characterized by long, slow, deep inhalation and exhalation. Emphysema patients tend to breathe in a shallow, rapid manner, relying primarily on their chest muscles. This short, rapid respiration not only fails to allow sufficient passage of air through the lungs but also tends to produce tension and fatigue in the chest muscles. Abdominal breathing helps eliminate these problems and at the same time facilitates the exchange of oxygen and carbon dioxide.

The best position for learning how to do abdominal breathing is lying on your back. Place both of your hands on your abdomen. Then consciously breathe in and out slowly and deeply in a relaxed manner.

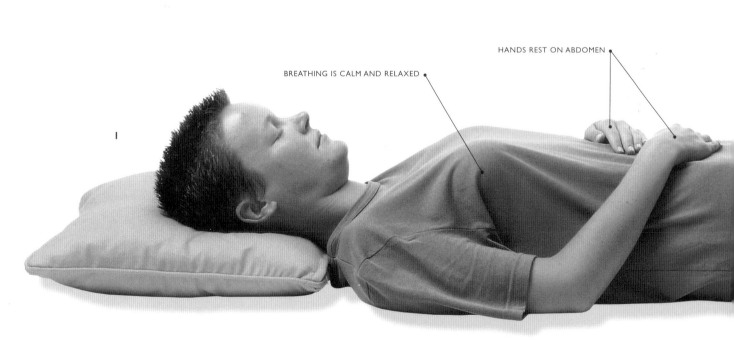

HANDS REST ON ABDOMEN

BREATHING IS CALM AND RELAXED

1

In addition, breathing exercises help reduce muscle tension and relax both the body and mind. Before starting relaxation exercises, patients should warm up with breathing exercises. A combination of the two types of exercise will produce the most effective relief of tension. Last but not least, following breathing routines also clears out phlegm, freeing the air passages from any obstruction.

Breathing exercises for those who are suffering from pulmonary emphysema focus on abdominal breathing, which makes breathing out easier. Abdominal breathing depends on contraction between the abdominal muscles and the diaphragm. During inhalation, the diaphragm expands and moves downward, thereby creating a pressure that forces the abdominal cavity to rise and the chest cavity to enlarge. The opposite effects occur during the process of exhalation. The diaphragm moves upward to its original position and the abdomen falls.

Abdominal breathing can be mixed with other kinds of exercises. It can also be performed using the methods of Chi Kung, especially Chiang Chuang Kung, or invigorating breathing (*see pp. 74–77*). Abdominal breathing should be practiced 2 or 3 times a day for sessions of 10 to 20 minutes to help develop new breathing techniques.

2 **Focus on your abdomen and try to make the air you breathe go all the way to the abdomen. As you inhale, you will feel the abdomen rise. It will fall as you exhale.**

2

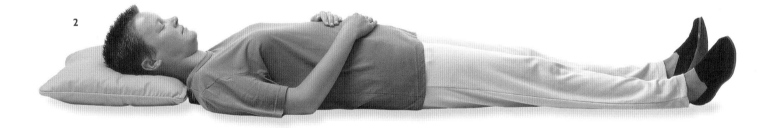

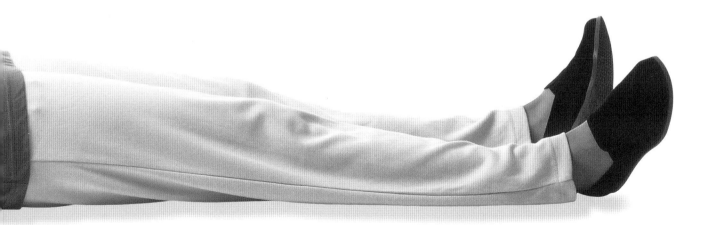

Practice the following exhalation exercises twice a day for 5 to 10 minutes. To avoid light-headedness, limit the number of repetitions in each series to a comfortable level. To achieve the best results from these healing exercises, they should be performed only after the inflammation in the respiratory tract is under control. And they should be practiced with regularity and persistence. Their ultimate purpose is to help the patient develop the habit of breathing abdominally at all times.

SET 1 ▮ String blowing

Hang a piece of string about 18in (46cm) from your face. Sit on a chair with your back straight and do not lean forward. Exhale strongly to make the string blow in the wind. As you get better at this, you can move the string (or yourself) farther and farther away.

SET 2 ▮ Blowing bubbles

With a straw, blow bubbles in a glass of water. Try to make bubbles for as long as possible, and endeavor to make the bubbling last a little longer each day.

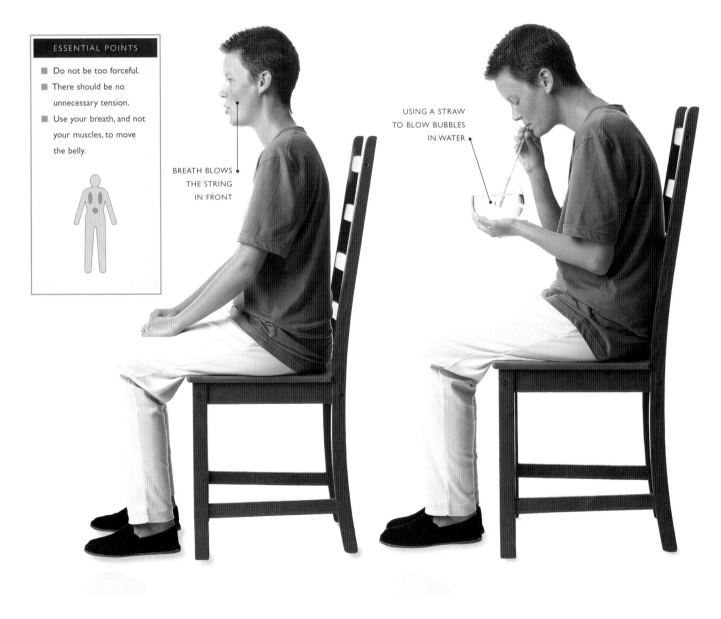

ESSENTIAL POINTS

- Do not be too forceful.
- There should be no unnecessary tension.
- Use your breath, and not your muscles, to move the belly.

BREATH BLOWS
THE STRING
IN FRONT

USING A STRAW
TO BLOW BUBBLES
IN WATER

SET 3 ‖ Extended exhalation

Stand with your hands resting lightly on your hips. Breathe deeply, letting the exhalation take more than twice the amount of time required for inhalation. Breathe in through the nose, but breathe out through **the mouth with your lips rounded into a whistling shape. Let the air come out through the opening between upper and lower teeth or through the pursed lips. Remember to use abdominal breathing.**

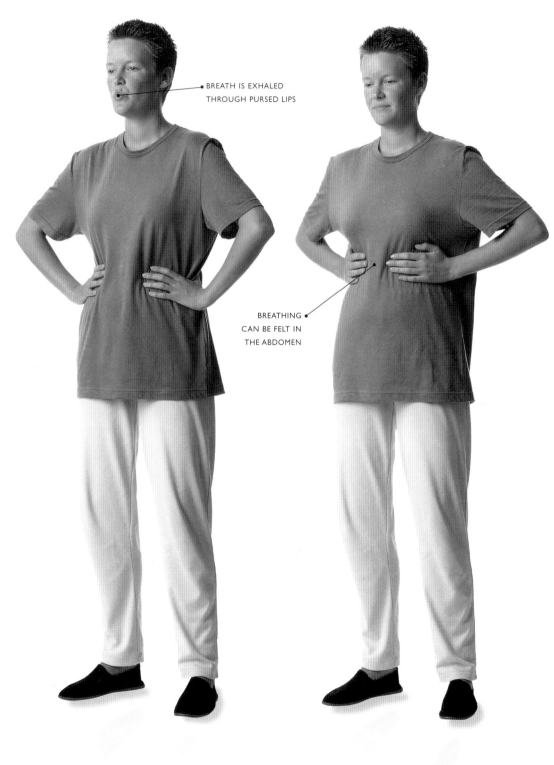

BREATH IS EXHALED
THROUGH PURSED LIPS

BREATHING
CAN BE FELT IN
THE ABDOMEN

SET 4 | Feeling the breath

Stand with your hands against the sides of your waist as you breathe in through your nose. While breathing out through your mouth, move your hands up and press them against the sides of your chest to aid in expelling the air.

SET 5 | Twisting

Sit on a stool, with your back straight. Lace your fingers behind your neck. Slowly rotate your upper body from the waist, turning first to the left, then to the right. This exercise is designed to strengthen the joints between your ribs and vertebrae so that you can breathe more slowly and deeply. The movement should be slow and steady. Reduce the speed if you feel dizzy.

ARMS TWIST
ALTERNATELY TO
LEFT AND RIGHT

HANDS HELP PUSH
OUT THE AIR

ESSENTIAL POINTS

- Feel the breath moving the abdomen.
- Keep your shoulders and arms relaxed—there should be no unnecessary muscle tension.

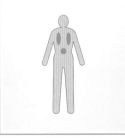

SET 6 ▮ Squeezing air out

Stand with your arms spread out to the sides while you inhale through your nose. While exhaling through your nose, squeeze your forearms against your upper abdomen to help the air come out.

SET 7 ▮ Squatting

Stand with your feet shoulder-width apart, your arms hanging loosely by your sides. Breathe in deeply while lifting your head slightly upward. Then breathe out deeply while squatting down with both hands pressed firmly against the abdomen.

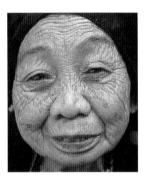

Healing Exercise and Elderly Bronchitis Patients

Many older patients who have chronic bronchitis also have some degree of emphysema, but they too can be helped by therapeutic exercise. Even if bronchitis patients have no trace of pulmonary emphysema, they should practice healing exercise to improve their overall fitness, enhance their lung function, and help avoid acute attacks of tracheitis.

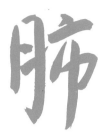

■ **Old age should not be a barrier to undertaking gentle exercise.**

By combining medication with healing exercise, Chinese doctors in recent years have made significant progress in preventing chronic bronchitis. And it has been found that patients who persistently practiced their exercises over a long period caught fewer colds. They also improved their lung capacity, their ability to take in oxygen and the strength of their diaphragm. Shortness of breath and chest discomfort—common symptoms of chronic bronchitis—were also relieved.

The therapeutic exercises for treating chronic bronchitis in the elderly are basically the same as those used to treat pulmonary emphysema (*see pp. 132–137*), but they also include a massage for preventing colds (*see pp. 124–125*) as well as cold-water tolerance training.

Chinese doctors have found that cold-water tolerance training can help prevent bronchitis attacks and colds as well as increase tolerance to cold temperatures. Starting in the summer, so that it comes as less of a shock to your system, begin washing your face with cold water, making sure you do not miss the nose. Repeat this washing every morning, continuing right into the winter. When the weather is warm, you can also rub cold water over your chest, or even over the whole body if you feel you can bear this.

If you have chronic bronchitis but are sufficiently strong, then rapid walking, walking up and down stairs (*see pp. 130–131*), jogging, hiking, Tai Chi (*see pp. 60–67*), or any simple callisthenic program can be beneficial. You should try to exercise outdoors and make sure that you get plenty of fresh air.

If you have a lot of phlegm, proper posture, combined with exercise therapy such as physiotherapy or chest massage (*see pp. 128–129*), can help get rid of it. You need to lie on your side with a firm pillow under your lower chest so that your body arches over it. The physiotherapist will then massage your chest and tap on your back at the same time to help loosen the phlegm and let it be expelled as you cough. This process will take 5 or 10 minutes. At home, you could ask someone

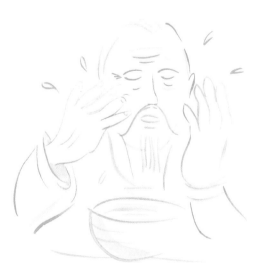

■ **Splashing the face with cold water is seen as a good way to help prevent colds and attacks of bronchitis.**

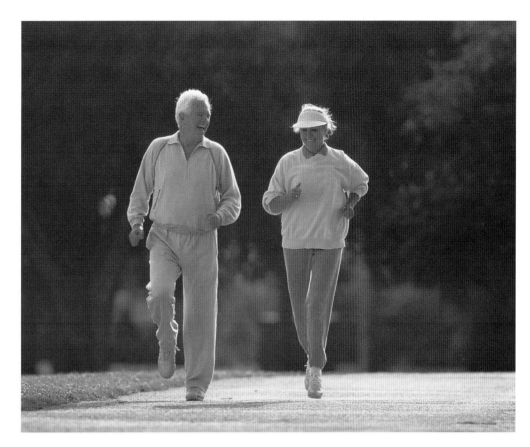

to tap your back while you simultaneously massage your own chest.

Acupuncture, traditional Chinese medicine, and Tai Chi, combined with Chi Kung, have all been shown to be successful in the treatment of chronic bronchitis. The Up and Down Gymnastic Breathing Exercise (*see pp. 80–81*) and Hand Swinging or Li Shou (*see pp. 86–89*) are both specified as being beneficial exercises for this complaint.

■ **Even the elderly can enjoy a gentle jog in the park, provided their condition and their doctor permit it.**

In addition, dressing appropriately for the season and eating properly will also help. For instance, in order to counteract fluid retention you should limit your salt intake and eat more of the diuretic foods that are known to increase urinary output, such as celery, parsley, and dandelion leaves. Herbs like rosemary, cloves, thyme, and cinnamon are renowned as decongestants, so adding more of these to your food may well ease chest congestion.

■ **Physiotherapy can bring great relief by loosening excess phlegm, which can then be expelled by coughing.**

Exercise and Bronchial Asthma

Many asthma patients wonder if healing exercise can relieve a disease that is as hard to treat as bronchial asthma. However, in a study done outside China, doctors reported that 70 percent of patients who did healing exercise had decreased asthma symptoms. The same is true for asthma as for other complaints—if the body is in good general condition, the lungs will heal more quickly.

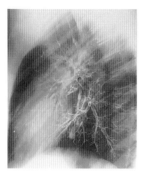

■ **When the lungs are healthy, the bronchial tree shows clearly on an X-ray.**

Though generally speaking it may not be easy to treat bronchial asthma, with proper exercise it is possible to decrease the frequency of attacks and to alleviate symptoms when they do occur. Performing special breathing exercises before or at the beginning of an asthma attack can prevent it from getting worse or can reduce its duration.

People with asthma tend to have a limited vital capacity, and their lungs may have deteriorated, with a tendency toward emphysema. Healing exercise can strengthen respiratory muscles, including those of the chest and diaphragm, and improve oxygen-carbon dioxide exchange. It can also reduce the incidence of bronchial spasms and improve blood circulation in the lungs. The mucus inside the bronchioles becomes thinner and easier to expel, and the symptoms are relieved. Therapeutic exercises for bronchial asthma patients include pronunciation breathing exercises, corrective breathing, relaxation exercises, massage, and Chi Kung.

CHEST SHOULD BE LOOSE AND RELAXED

SPINE IS STRAIGHT AND VERTICAL

HANDS SIT NATURALLY IN THE LAP

■ **Breathing and relaxation exercises may be performed from a sitting position if this is easier.**

CORRECTIVE BREATHING

These methods are the same as those for pulmonary emphysema. The aim is to develop the habit of breathing with the abdomen (*see pp. 132–133*) and to strengthen and prolong the process of exhaling (*see pp. 134–137*).

PRONUNCIATION BREATHING

Pronouncing words during exhalation helps instil a new way of breathing by associating breathing with sound. This exercise can be done while either sitting or standing. As you exhale through your mouth, pronounce the syllables "wu," "ee," and "ah." At first, hold each syllable for only 5 or 6 seconds. But after practicing for a while you can gradually increase the duration to 30 or 40 seconds. Take a break when you need one—you should not become fatigued.

■ **Young asthma sufferers may greatly improve the effectiveness of their breathing, and reduce their need for inhalers, by doing healing exercises.**

CHI KUNG

Both Fang Sung Kung, relaxation breathing (*see pp. 72–73*), and Chiang Chuang Kung, invigorating breathing (*see pp. 74–77*), are good for patients suffering from bronchial asthma. Sessions of 20 to 30 minutes once or twice a day will be beneficial.

The best physical fitness exercise for asthma patients is swimming, as it has been known to reduce the incidence of bronchial spasm. Patients with allergic rhinitis (hay fever) or recurrent ear infections should not dive or swim under the water, however.

Games that take from 1 to 2 minutes of playing time such as table tennis, badminton, or shooting basketballs are also good for asthmatics as they help reduce the chance of obstruction in the respiratory tract. The worse the condition appears before practice, the greater the degree of improvement in clearing the respiratory tract after 1 to 2 minutes of exercise.

Precautions for asthmatics doing healing exercise

✱ Only do healing exercise when you are free of an asthma attack or when the attack is very mild.

✱ Do not exercise rigorously for more than 5 minutes at a time unless your condition is well under control. More exercising might aggravate the condition, but brief strenuous exercises lasting 1 to 2 minutes may help reduce obstruction in the respiratory tract.

✱ If you experience chest discomfort or shortness of breath during practice, stop exercising and rest.

✱ If asthma attacks recur frequently and you are not making any gains in fitness, then stop exercising.

✱ Before exercising, blow your nose to clear out mucus.

✱ Exercise time should not exceed 30 to 40 minutes divided into 3 or 4 sessions. For example, do Chi Kung for 20 minutes, self-massage for 3 to 5 minutes, pronunciation exercises—with rest periods—for 3 to 5 minutes, and relaxation exercises for 1 to 2 minutes. One or two sets of abdominal breathing exercises may also be included.

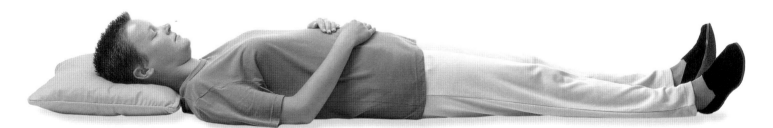

SET 1 | Relaxation exercise

Stand with your feet shoulder-width apart and your arms hanging loosely at your sides. Turn your body to the side, letting the shoulders turn naturally. Do this 10 times. You can also rotate your shoulders backward and forward, concentrating on letting the shoulder joints relax completely.

SET 2 | Relaxation exercise

Sit on a chair and bend your arms into a circle in front of you. Let your shoulder joints relax completely. Swing the circle to the left about 10 times, then to the right.

ESSENTIAL POINTS

- Let the shoulders be as relaxed as possible.
- There should be no unnecessary tension anywhere in the body.

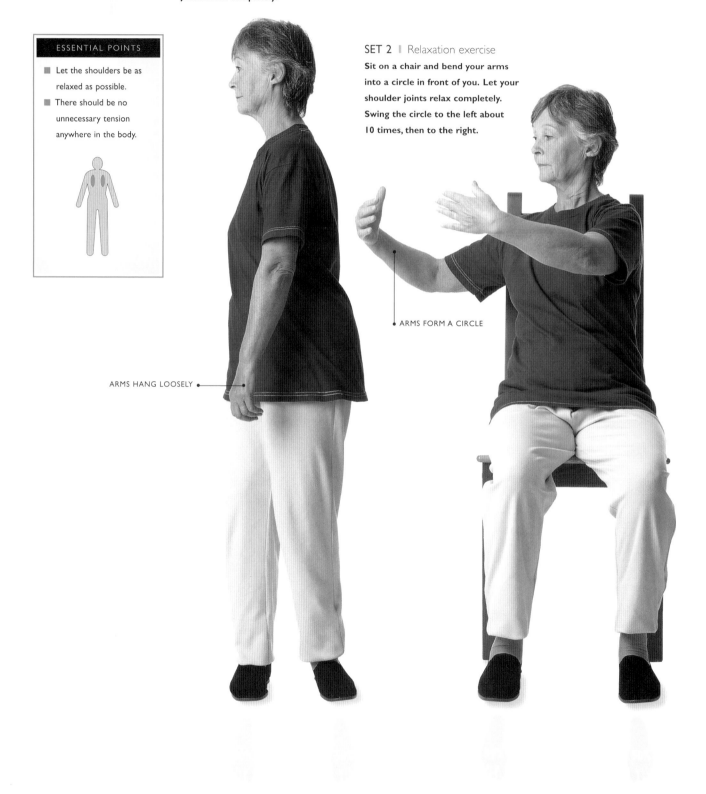

ARMS FORM A CIRCLE

ARMS HANG LOOSELY

SET 3 ‖ Massage

To help relieve discomfort in the chest and back region, try massage, which you can either do yourself or have done by a health professional. Massage the muscles that cover your ribs by pushing and rubbing the chest area.

Tap your back by bending over and getting someone to beat you on the back around the kidneys with a loose fist; the kidneys are believed to support the lungs. There is no limit to the number of times you can do this, as long as it feels comfortable.

HANDS MASSAGE •
THE CHEST

HANDS TAP THE BACK,
NEAR THE KIDNEYS •

肺

19

YUN DONG YU FA CHEN AI CHEN ZHEN BING BING REN

Exercise and Silicosis Patients

Silicosis is a common form of lung disease that is frequently found in miners and in metal and foundry workers. It is caused by inhaling silica, the particles of which irritate the lung tissues, impairing not only breathing but also general health. The patient then becomes more susceptible to tuberculosis.

As part of a comprehensive program for the treatment of silicosis, therapeutic exercise can contribute to improved breathing and health.

Symptoms such as coughing, panting, and chest pain are lessened, and the patient's ability to use oxygen and take in and expel air get better. Therapeutic exercises for silicosis patients consist mainly of breathing exercises, Tai Chi (*see pp. 60–67*) combined with Chi Kung breathing, callisthenics and similar routines.

Breathing exercises are intended to increase the diameter of the diaphragm and to extend the time that is spent exhaling. In addition to abdominal breathing (*see pp. 132–133*), useful breathing exercises include those that call for pressure to the abdomen or lower chest (*see pp. 136–137*).

Silicosis patients can also do relaxation exercises and a combination of physical and breathing exercises such as the following bellows technique.

ESSENTIAL POINTS

- Let the movement create the breathing.
- There should be no unnecessary tension in your body.

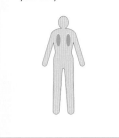

1 Sit on the side of a bed or on a chair with your buttocks near the edge of the seat. Open your legs wide and stretch both feet out in front of you. Rest your palms on your abdomen.

2 Breathe in deeply. Then bend the upper part of your body forward until your head is lower than your knees as you simultaneously press both hands against the abdomen in order to help move the diaphragm upward, exhaling as fully as possible.

● *Repeat the first three steps 7 to 14 times, before marching on the spot.*

1

2

Standing breathing posture

Stand with your feet shoulder-width or a bit wider apart and bend your knees slightly while keeping your back straight. Hold your chin up slightly and naturally, relax your shoulders and waist, and lift your arms, with the palms up. The thumbs should be slightly separate to activate the lung meridian. Breathe in lightly through your nose and out heavily through your mouth. The time spent inhaling is short; that spent exhaling is long. Make your breathing natural and without the slightest effort.

3 **Then relax both hands, raise your head and stretch your neck to the front while inhaling deeply as you slowly lift your body to the original position. By the time you are sitting up straight, you should have finished inhaling.**

4 **Finally, stand and march on the spot for 1 or 2 minutes. Then do 7 or 8 full squats to complete this exercise.**

3

4

100%

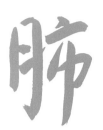

YUN DONG SHI RU HE DUI YING XIONG BU BU SHI

Combating Chest Pain while Exercising

It sometimes happens that patients with serious respiratory problems experience chest pain during physical activity. The symptoms may include pain that intensifies with conversation, breathing, or coughing. A crushing type of pain may also occur at times, although an X-ray and consultation with your doctor reveals no swelling, bruiselike hemorrhages, fractures, or any other abnormalities.

There are several possible causes of the pain (*see box opposite*), all of which can be easily rectified. However, if the pain seems serious, of course you should see a doctor. Otherwise, there are some simple techniques that may help to relieve your chest pain.

As simple a thing as lying down and rolling around in bed may also do the trick and relieve your pain.

ESSENTIAL POINTS

Relaxing the body is the key to good health. Use your breathing, and not muscle tension, to work the lungs.

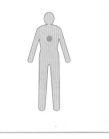

Try taking a deep breath and holding it as you knock on your chest from top to bottom using a loose fist. Repeat this several times or until the pain stops.

FISTS KNOCK ON CHEST

BODY IS HELD LOOSELY

Get someone else to pound the side and back of your chest from top to bottom, using a loose fist. Repeat this several times, or until the pain stops.

FISTS POUND
BACK AND SIDE

Possible causes of pain

✱ You may not have warmed up sufficiently, moving straight into physically demanding exercise without adequate preparatory work.

✱ You may have neglected your deep breathing during your workout, and been breathing in and out without rhythm.

✱ The rate of your breathing may have been so rapid that you were not able to get enough oxygen.

✱ Your respiratory muscles may have been too tense for too long.

✱ You may have started with a body that was overtaxed and weak.

✱ You may not have done any form of exercise for a long time.

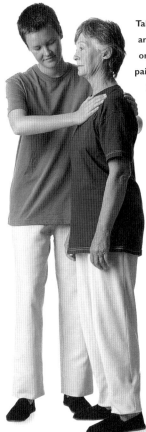

Take several deep breaths and then press your hand on the painful spot. The pain will usually go away. If someone else is doing this, have the person place one hand on the painful spot and the other opposite it on the back. The palms can then massage and press from both sides.

CHAPTER FIVE

Improving your digestion by means of healing exercise

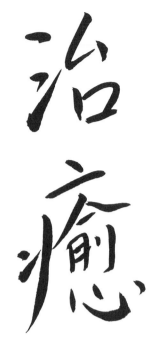

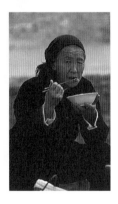

■ **The Chinese have traditionally treated the digestive system with respect.**

Sayings and lore in all cultures (such as "You are what you eat") testify to the importance that human beings accord to their digestive tracts. The Chinese, however, grant even more dignity and meaning to this system, and treat it with the appropriate respect. This chapter looks at some of the successful ways that the Chinese have developed to heal digestive complaints—from common problems such as constipation and hemorrhoids to more serious illnesses such as ulcers and gall stones.

The digestive system begins with cooking, which breaks food down; chewing and stomach acids then continue the process, and nutrients are extracted to form blood to heal the body. The digestive process continues in the small and large intestines, and then waste is excreted. All processes must be working effectively for the body to be in good health. The Chinese have developed numerous exercises to aid the digestion of food, the absorption of nutrients and the excretion of waste, so that the body can stay healthy and strong.

■ **Drinking copious amounts of water helps to nourish the body and hydrate the skin.**

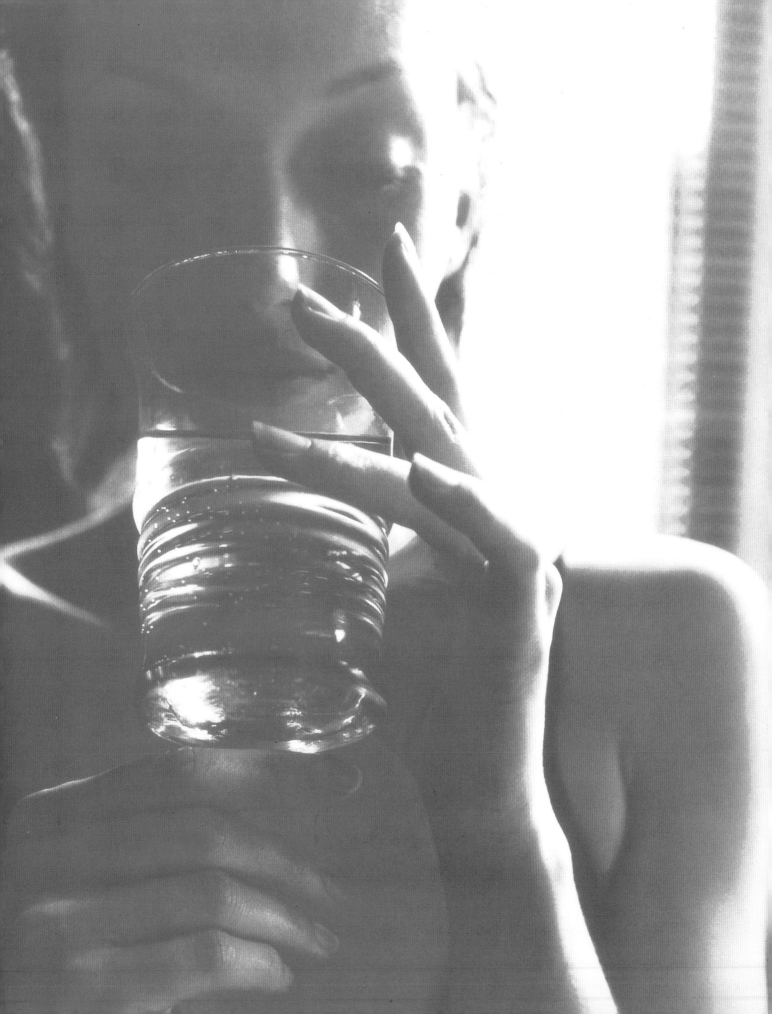

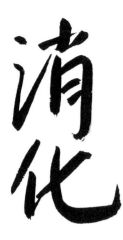

21

ZHI LIAO BIAN BI

Curing Constipation

Changes in eating habits and bowel schedules are often cited as reasons for constipation. In fact, the most common cause of habitual constipation is physical inactivity. The best way to prevent or eliminate constipation is to exercise frequently, maintain a fixed bowel routine, and watch your diet. You should eat plenty of green vegetables and fresh fruit, as well as whole grains, bran, lentils, and beans. You should also drink plenty of fresh water—at least eight glasses a day. A small amount of honey may be helpful, too.

SET 1 | Leg bending

1 **Lie on your back with your legs out straight.**

ESSENTIAL POINTS

- The main emphasis in leg bending is on the belly, so relax both your shoulders and your neck.
- If you feel that the back is being strained, ease off the exercise.

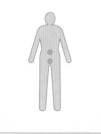

2 **Bend your legs, raise them, and draw them in to touch your abdomen. Return to the starting position. Repeat 10 or more times.**

SET 2 | Pretend pedaling

Lie on your back, lift your legs into the air, and pretend to pedal a bicycle. Your movements should be relatively quick, rhythmical, and smooth. Perform this exercise in 20- to 30-second bursts.

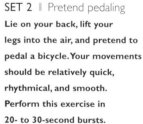
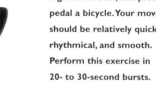

Therapeutic exercise

Therapeutic exercises, particularly those involving the abdomen and waist and those requiring jumping and deep breathing, can stimulate intestinal movement (thereby relieving constipation); they can also strengthen the abdominal muscles and have beneficial effects on the nervous system. The latter effect in itself helps prevent constipation. People who suffer from habitual constipation can benefit most from therapeutic gymnastics, exercise therapy, Chi Kung, Tai Chi, and self-massage.

As with all therapeutic gymnastics, the following exercises should be performed in a specific order to achieve the maximum benefit.

SET 3 ‖ Leg lifting

1 **Lie on your back with your legs out straight.** Lift both of your legs simultaneously, without bending your knees.

2 **Raise the legs until they are perpendicular to your body.** Then slowly lower them, keeping your knees straight. Repeat 10 or more times.

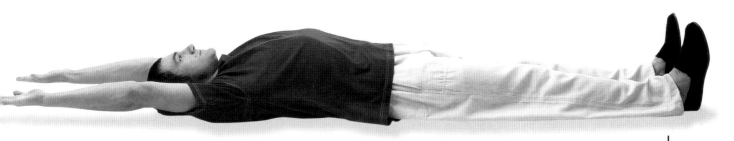

SET 4 ‖ Sit-ups

1 **Start on your back with your legs straight out and your arms over your head.**

2 **Do sit-ups, reaching all the way down to touch the tips of your toes. Do this 7 or 8 times. (If it is too difficult or hurts your back, you can do partial sit-ups with knees bent and arms at your side.)**

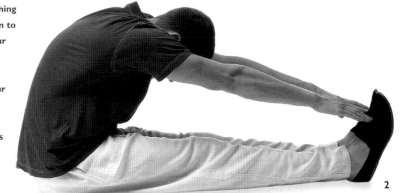

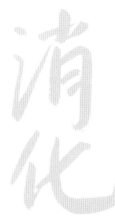

Exercise therapy

The most effective exercises are walking, jogging, and canoeing. The best time to walk is in the early morning. Immediately after getting up, walk outside at a fast pace for 30 minutes. If you are physically weak, you can take a leisurely walk for about 15 minutes after breakfast—if your doctor agrees. Afterward, drink a glass of water and then attempt to move your bowels. A regular outdoor walk of 1½–2 miles (2.5–3.2km) is also recommended any time during the day.

The vibrations that are produced by running and jumping also have a stimulating effect on the intestines and facilitate bowel movements. People who are physically fit may jog, play basketball, and do similar exercises. The rowing motion in canoeing can also help to stimulate intestinal movement.

Chi Kung

Nei Yang Kung, internally nourishing breathing (*see pp. 78–79*), is recommended for people with constipation problems. Perform these abdominal breathing exercises in a lying-down or sitting position for 30 minutes or so, 2 or 3 times a day.

Chi Kung works to prevent or treat constipation because it improves your emotional state. It also restores the proper balance between sympathetic nervous system inhibition and stimulation, which is vital to normal bowel functioning. And during deep abdominal breathing, the diaphragm moves up and down rhythmically massaging both the stomach and intestine. During abdominal breathing, the activity of the diaphragm is 3 to 4 times greater than normal. If someone were to put an ear to your abdomen, the results of Chi Kung would be clearly audible.

ESSENTIAL POINTS

■ For best results you should combine Tai Chi with Chi Kung breathing techniques.

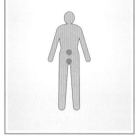

SHOULDERS ARE LOOSE AND RELAXED

BREATH IS DRAWN IN THROUGH THE NOSE, USING THE ABDOMINAL METHOD

Massage

Gentle massage of the abdomen can help heal bowel ailments. The entire sequence counts as one circle. Do this 30 to 40 times. If you prefer, you may massage by the clock for, say, 10 minutes. After your abdominal massage, sit down and lightly tap the sacrum (the hard area in the small of your back). This massage may be performed once or twice a day. It is particularly good after therapeutic gymnastics or Chi Kung.

While lying flat on your back with your legs bent slightly and your knees supported by a pillow, perform self-massage by pushing and pressing down on the abdominal region with one hand positioned on top of the other. Start the massage on the lower right side of the abdomen, then move up to the rib area. Continue in a circular motion, moving to the left side, crossing over the navel, and rubbing until the hands reach the lower left side of the abdomen. Rub and press against this area slowly but deeply, before returning to the original position.

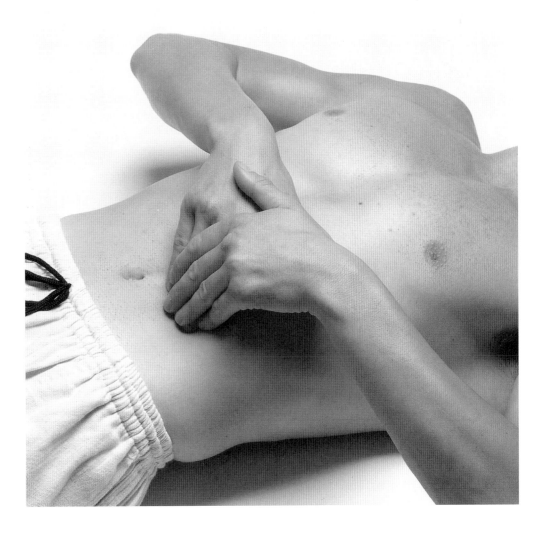

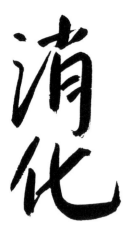

(22)

AN MA GAI SHAN XIAN HUA BU LIANG

Relieving Indigestion with Massage

When the digestive system is not functioning well, belching, nausea, vomiting, abdominal pain, and gas often occur. Massaging the abdomen can help alleviate these symptoms. The use of massage as both a preventive and a healing technique has a long history in Chinese medicine. One ancient medical text says that "indigestion can be relieved by first massaging the abdomen with both hands and then walking a distance of one hundred steps." The same book mentions that "massaging the abdomen after a meal can aid the functioning of the spleen and prevent indigestion."

Studies have shown that massaging the abdominal region not only heightens the level of activity in the stomach and intestines but also promotes circulation in the abdominal cavity. Massaging the acupuncture points that relate to the abdomen can also help (*see pp. 166–167*).

Massage for indigestion

A session of massaging the abdomen should last for about 20 minutes. You can either perform the massage yourself or have someone else do it for you, which may be more relaxing.

ESSENTIAL POINTS

- Just before doing the massage rub your hands until they are warm.
- Imagine healing *chi* energy flowing from the hands during the massage.

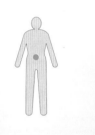

SET 1 | Massaging the abdomen

1 Rub the palm of your hand on your upper left abdomen. If this region is distended due to the presence of gas, perform the massage with a vibrating finger motion.

2 Move to the lower right abdomen and massage in a circular motion around your navel, moving up from the bottom and from the right to the left. A small amount of pressure can be applied while you are rubbing.

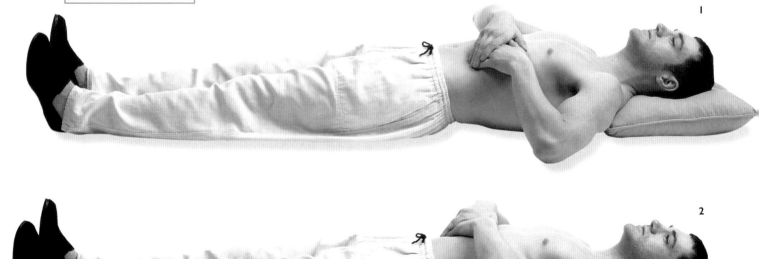

Strengthening the muscles of the abdominal wall

Many middle-aged people and women after pregnancy have a slack abdominal wall, which can cause the abdomen to become distended and large and to hang forward and down. Weak and loose abdominal muscles are responsible. Sometimes, excessive fat that is deposited in the abdominal wall aggravates the problem, as well as hampering blood circulation and impeding digestive functions.

If uncorrected, a slack abdominal wall can lead to other ailments. For example, those who have a slack abdominal wall are likely to develop constipation—their abdominal muscles are simply too weak to contract properly, and the abdominal wall cannot exert enough pressure to move the bowel. Tai Chi done in combination with Chi Kung strengthens the belly.

Another problem created by an out-of-shape abdomen is that the body is forced to adjust its center of gravity. To compensate for the distended abdomen, the lumbar vertebrae turn forward, creating strain on back muscles. This is why people with slack abdominal walls are more likely to suffer from lumbago or lower back pain (*see pp. 198–201*) as well.

To correct a slack abdominal wall, you can strengthen the abdominal muscles alone or do exercises to improve the body as a whole. These are particularly important for people who are overweight, because whole-body exercises use up more energy and have a greater impact on cutting down the amount of fat stored. The therapeutic gymnastics that are recommended for constipation (*see pp. 150–151*) are excellent for strengthening the abdomen.

SET 2 ❚ Scissor kicks

1 Lie on your back and raise your legs about 45 degrees from the ground. Keep the small of your back pressed to the floor.

2 Do scissor kicks in the air until your legs tire. Rest for a minute, then repeat the kicks 3 to 4 times.

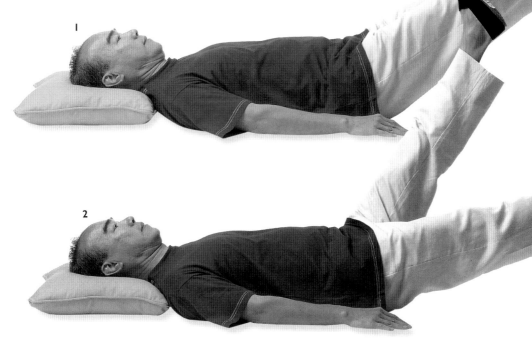

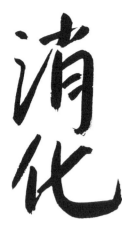

(23)

FANG ZHI ZHI JI

Preventing Hemorrhoids

Habitual constipation, poor eating habits— including indulging in foods with strong spices—persistent diarrhea or dysentery, chronic stomach and intestine diseases, aging, and a generally weakened body and slack muscles are some of the primary causes of hemorrhoids. Other contributory factors may be: a rise in the pressure of the portal veins; cirrhosis; an increase in the pressure in the abdomen caused by pregnancy or tumors; high blood pressure; arteriosclerosis; or chronic inflammation of the rectum.

Perhaps the most important factor is simply that humans walk on two feet instead of on four —animals that walk on four feet do not get hemorrhoids because their pelvic cavities do not have to support their abdominal organs. Blood circulation is also significant in this respect. The return of venous blood to the heart relies on muscle contraction and the functioning of valves

SET 1 ▌ Inner thigh squeeze

Lie on your back in a relaxed position and cross one leg over the other, letting it rest there. Then press your inner thighs together while at the same time tightening and lifting your anus. Repeat this squeeze 10 to 30 times. As you become accustomed to this exercise, you can also combine it with breathing techniques, inhaling deeply as you squeeze and exhaling as you relax.

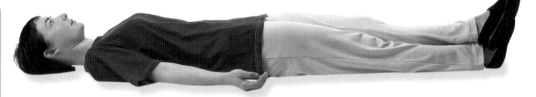

ESSENTIAL POINTS

■ Gradually combine the exercises with breathing techniques as you become more proficient.

■ The tightening of the anus should create a feeling of pulling inward and upward.

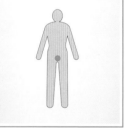

SET 2 ▌ Arm raising

1 **Lie on your back with your arms resting beside your body. Relax.**

2 **Without bending your elbows, raise your arms up, back and over your head as you breathe in deeply. Exhale as you bring your arms back to your sides. Repeat 5 to 6 times.**

1

2a

inside the veins. The valves make sure that the blood in the veins can flow only in the direction of the heart and never away from the heart. To prevent the flow of blood in the wrong direction, human beings are equipped with valves in veins below the level of the heart, but not in the rectal veins because evolutionary design intended the rectum to be on the same level as the heart when they walked. As a result, blood can back up in these vessels and pressure caused by gravity, strain, or other factors can cause them to distend into hemorrhoids.

The following nine exercises can have healing benefits for hemorrhoid sufferers. You can expect to see results in 3 months if you practice them 1 to 3 times a day. If time is a problem, do only three exercises: inner thigh squeeze, crossed-leg sitting and standing, and squeeze and relax.

Once the condition has been brought under control, you can practice the anal constriction exercises to speed recovery. These exercises should be practiced regularly, with gradually increasing intensity, in order to achieve the maximum benefit.

SET 3 ▌ Pelvic lift

1 **Lie on your back with your knees bent, feet flat on the floor, and your hands under your head.**

2 **Raise your pelvis off the floor, while simultaneously lifting and constricting your anus. Then lower your pelvis and relax the anus. After a while, start practicing constricting your anus as you breathe in and relaxing it as you breathe out. Work up to 8 repetitions.**

SET 4 ▌ Self-massage

Place your hand over your abdomen so that Chi Hai (The Sea of Chi), which is located about 1½in (3.75cm) below the navel, is in the center. Rub your abdominal muscles, first in a counterclockwise direction for 20 to 30 circles, then in a clockwise direction for 20 to 30 circles.

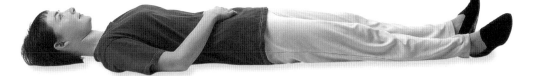

2b

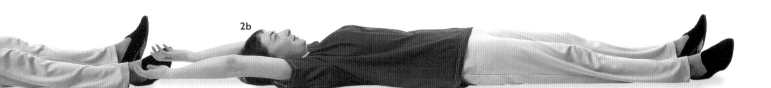

SET 5 | Crossed-leg sitting and standing

| Sit on the floor with your legs crossed. **Relax your entire body.**

2 Stand up, keeping your legs crossed and pressed tightly against each other, while constricting your anus. Keeping your legs crossed, sit down again and relax completely. Repeat 10 to 30 times.

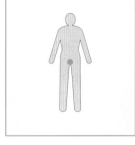

1

2

SET 6 | Squeeze and relax

| Stand with your legs crossed and pressed tightly against each other, while also constricting your anus.

2 Without uncrossing your legs, relax your body as much as possible. Do this squeeze-and-relax sequence 20 to 50 times, depending on your own physical condition.

1

2

SET 7 | Abdominal knock

Stand with your legs crossed. Inhale as you press your legs against each other and tighten your anus. After a full inhalation, breathe out while knocking lightly against your abdomen with loose fists. Repeat the tightening and knocking sequence 20 to 40 times. Increase the force of the knock gradually and cautiously. If you feel discomfort in your abdomen, reduce the intensity.

SET 8 | Arm stretching on tiptoe

Stand with your feet close together and arms naturally by your sides. Stretch your arms over your head and rise up on your toes as you inhale deeply. Exhale as you return to the starting position. Repeat 5 to 6 times.

SET 9 | Bowing with arms back

Stand with your feet shoulder-width apart. Make loose fists and lift them to the sides of your chest at nipple level as you breathe in. Keep your elbows back, your chest open, and your head up.

2 **As you exhale, bend gracefully forward into a deep bow with hands stretched backward and up, and your palms open. Repeat 5 to 6 times.**

1

2

(24)

YU FANG ZHI CHANG XIA CHUI

Exercises for Rectal Prolapse
and the Intestines

A prolapse of the anus happens when the mucous membranes that line the rectum are displaced downward. The internal mucous membranes detach from the underlying wall and protrude from the anus.

Rectal prolapse may be caused by a number of factors. In young patients, the ligaments and muscles that make up the pelvic floor may not have developed enough to be able to give proper support to the rectum. Poor health in general, malnutrition, or recurrent diarrhea can also contribute to this condition. In elderly patients, rectal prolapse may be caused by a combination of poor health, slack muscles and ligaments, and gravity's pull on the stomach and intestines. Frequent childbirth in women who are not physically fit can cause the muscles that support the rectum to become slack. A chronic cough or abdominal pressure from other sources can also cause a prolapse of the rectum. Hemorrhoids, a slack sphincter muscle, or a rectal fissure are also contributory factors.

According to traditional Chinese medicine, prolapse of the rectum may be symptomatic of a number of underlying conditions. Chinese doctors believe that the most important causes of rectal prolapse are deficiencies in internal energy and blood. When these are in short supply, the body fails to absorb a sufficient amount of nutrients.

ESSENTIAL POINTS

■ Rub the hands together until they feel warm with *chi* just before beginning these massage techniques.

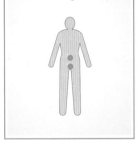

● *If done regularly, the pointed finger massage will not only alleviate stomach and intestine-related diseases but will also improve general health and encourage restful sleep.*

SET 1 ▌ Kneading the abdomen

Before getting up in the morning and just before going to bed, knead and rub around the navel with one hand in an anticlockwise direction. Using one hand, make 30 to 100 circles. Apply some pressure when kneading, but don't hurt yourself. Then make 30 to 100 clockwise circles with the other hand.

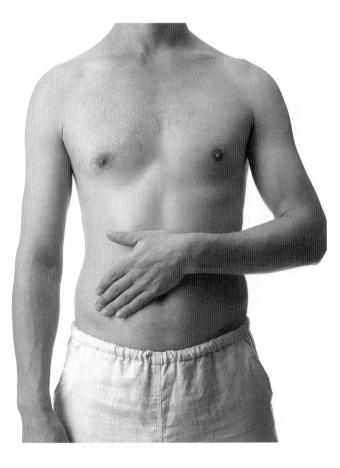

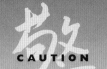

CAUTION

Do not perform these exercises after a heavy meal or if there is acute inflammation, a tumor, bleeding or high fever.

Chinese medicine recognizes a close connection between overall health and the condition of the perineum and the anus. Overall health can be improved through a conscious effort to keep the anus in good condition. Ancient medical specialists recommended frequent use of an exercise known as closing the gate, in which the anus is constricted. Many Chinese martial arts also emphasize the exercise of lifting the anus.

Just like muscles in the arms and legs, the muscles that make up the pelvic floor can be strengthened by exercise. And these exercises are effective in preventing prolapse of the anus. The same techniques designed for relieving hemorrhoids (*see pp. 156–159*) can be used for treating prolapse of the anus. However, patients with anal prolapse should practice the exercises mainly in a lying-down position. Before starting any exercise, the patient should push any protruding portion of the rectum back into its original position. The exercise should proceed gradually and cautiously. If acute inflammation occurs, it should be treated before resuming an exercise schedule.

Ulcers, an irritated stomach, fallen stomach, irritable bowel syndrome, and habitual constipation can also be treated by means of self-massage. Choose one of the two massage techniques described below, depending on which feels more comfortable to you.

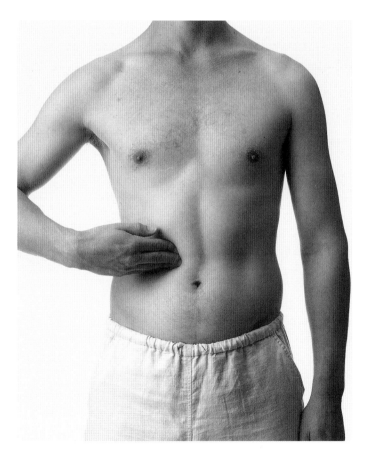

SET 2 | Pointed finger massage

Press down with your finger tips slowly but with some force at any spot on your abdomen. Press as deeply as possible without experiencing any pain, before releasing the fingers slowly. Press each spot deeply 3 to 5 times. Although you can start the pointed finger massage anywhere, it is best to begin at a spot on the upper abdomen. And it is best to follow a systematic pattern—moving around the edges and spiralling inward, for instance. Do the exercise for as long as feels comfortable to you.

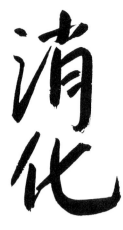

Healing Stomach and Intestinal Ulcers

To help the healing of both stomach and intestinal ulcers, try to avoid emotionally or psychologically stressful situations if at all possible, as these can make ulcers worse. You should also stop eating foods that will aggravate the condition, such as hot spices, strong curries, chili peppers and deep-fried food, as well as smoked and pickled foods.

> **CAUTION**
>
> If your condition is serious, you should postpone exercising until it has improved or stabilized— check with your doctor. Strenuous exercises may cause severe pain or even result in bleeding or stomach perforation.

Chi Kung has proved to be effective in treating gastric and duodenal ulcers (ulcers that occur in the stomach and upper part of the small intestine), largely because the mental quietness and tranquility that are associated with these exercises have an inhibitory effect on cortical activity—active thought processes. Overstimulation of the cerebral cortex in the brain —as a result of anxiety, nervousness, or extreme excitability— and the development of ulcers are closely related. A spirit of optimism can speed up the recovery process; anxiety and impatience may have an adverse effect.

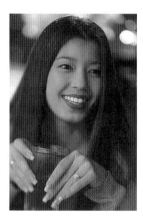

■ **Emotional state and diet are both strongly linked to the occurrence of stomach and intestinal ulcers.**

Both Nei Yang Kung, or internally nourishing breathing (*see pp. 78–79*), and Fang Sung Kung, or relaxation breathing (*see pp. 72–73*), are highly beneficial to ulcer patients. You should practice these techniques either lying on your side or sitting down. Do the exercises described in 30-minute sessions, 2 or 3 times a day.

In addition to Chi Kung, patients with stomach and intestinal ulcers may practice Tai Chi (*see pp. 60–67*) in order to gain considerable healing benefits. Abdominal massage (*see p. 153*) may also be therapeutic. It is important that a proper balance between activity and relaxation is maintained. Take care not to overdo strenuous exercise.

■ **Breathing techniques are all-important in the treatment of ulcers.**

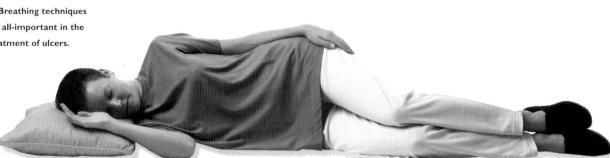

■ **Gentle walking is highly therapeutic for those with mild diabetes.**

HOW PHYSICAL EXERCISE CAN HELP DIABETES

Diabetes is a disease in which the pancreas does not make enough—or any—insulin, resulting in abnormally high levels of glucose, a simple sugar, in the blood. Physical exercise, diet, oral hypoglycemic agents, and insulin therapy are the major approaches to the treatment of diabetes used by most specialists. Exercise contributes to proper utilization of sugar by the body and has been shown to help reduce insulin consumption, improve the ability to breathe, reduce the pain in the joints, and relieve diabetes-related itching and constipation.

Healing exercise is most effective for patients who have relatively mild diabetes. Exercises frequently recommended include Chi Kung, Tai Chi, and leisurely walking.

Nei Yang Kung, internally nourishing breathing (*see pp. 78–79*), is the best form of Chi Kung for helping diabetics. Practice twice a day for about 30 minutes each time, in either the lying-down or the sitting position.

You should do Tai Chi once a day—either the complete set (*see pp. 62–67*) or simplified movements based on Tai Chi (*see pp. 60–61*), depending on your condition.

■ **Diabetics can benefit from the gentle arts of both Tai Chi and Chi Kung.**

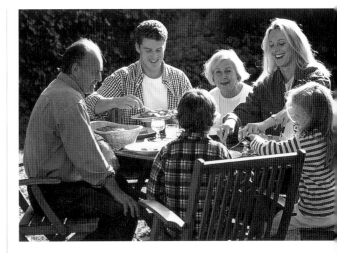

■ **Despite dietary restrictions and the need for insulin therapy, there is no reason why diabetics—aided by healing exercise—cannot live a normal family life.**

Leisurely walking after a meal—at a rate of just 2 miles (3.2km) an hour—can increase your rate of metabolism, helping your body to break down and digest the food you have just eaten. If you are in good shape, you can also go on hikes, canoe, or take part in similar activities. Choose according to your age, health, and personal preference.

Preventing Gall Bladder Disease by Diet and Exercise

One of the most common causes of gall bladder disease is a poor long-term diet. To prevent gall bladder problems occurring (prevention being always better than cure) you should avoid spicy and deep-fried foods and eat plenty of organic fruit and vegetables, together with whole-grain cereals, which can assist in eliminating cholesterol, a major component of gallstones.

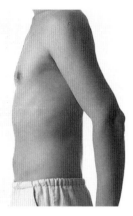

■ **People with gall bladder problems may experience discomfort in the abdomen after eating a big meal.**

The gall bladder is a small sac that stores bile manufactured in the liver; it is connected to the small intestine by the bile duct. Inflammation of the gall bladder may occur by itself, but it is usually accompanied by gallstones. A chronically inflamed gall bladder is one of the most frequent causes of digestive disorders. The patient often suffers from a bloated feeling, belching, constipation, and the inability to digest fatty foods. If you have gall bladder trouble, after a heavy meal you may feel discomfort in your upper abdomen. Pains in the lower corner of your shoulder blade and in the right side of your waist may occur often, particularly when you are doing standing exercise, or when you are bending or rising from a sitting position.

When the bile duct is obstructed—for example by thick, or sluggish, bile which may even have formed stones—an acutely inflamed gall bladder will result, often causing severe pain and jaundice. Thick bile may be associated with infection—which may be aggravated by the gallstones themselves—or with defective bile ducts, a chronically inflamed liver or even metabolic imbalances

Regular and systematic healing exercise, especially breathing exercise, stimulates the organs in the abdominal cavity and facilitates the secretion of bile. By keeping the system flowing, exercise can be an effective means of preventing gall bladder problems. It is particularly useful to

The gall bladder

The gall bladder is a pear-shaped sac, hidden by the liver and about 3¼in (8cm) long. When it is triggered by a hormone, it contracts, forcing bile into the cystic duct, the bile duct, and then the duodenum, where the bile breaks up fat globules.

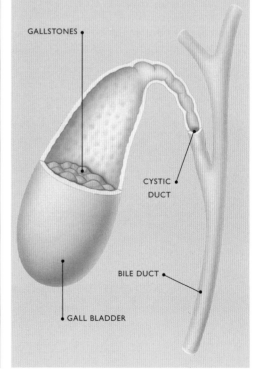

GALLSTONES

CYSTIC DUCT

BILE DUCT

GALL BLADDER

■ **The Chinese have long known of the benefits of Tai Chi for those suffering from gall bladder disease.**

■ **Rollerblading may be too extreme, but exercise of some sort is vital.**

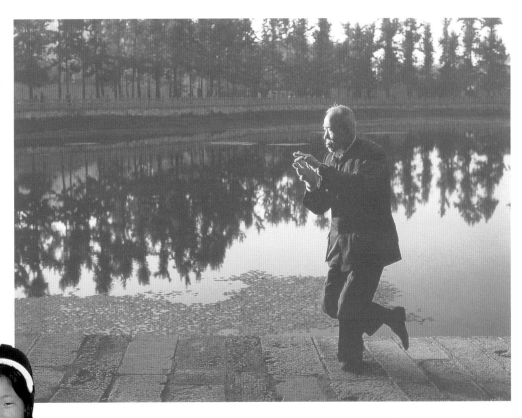

patients who are recovering from chronic liver inflammation.

Under certain conditions, exercise may not be appropriate. For example, in the case of repeated gall bladder infections coupled with other complications, surgical removal of the gall bladder may be the only option. Healing exercises are useful for treating gall bladder inflammation and gallstones when they have not yet reached the critical stage.

Based on your condition, your doctor may suggest that you choose from among the following exercises: walking, breathing exercises, Tai Chi, Chi Kung breathing exercise, and self-massage.

❋ **Walking:** Try taking a leisurely daily walk of 30 minutes or so. In the beginning, your pace should be slow and easy-going. When you feel better, you can increase your speed gradually.

❋ **Breathing exercises:** The breathing exercises that are suggested for silicosis patients (*see pp. 144–145*) are perfect.

❋ **Tai Chi:** You can practice the basic set (*see pp. 62–67*) from 1 to 3 times a day.

❋ **Chi Kung:** Follow the Nei Yang Kung technique of internally nourishing breathing (*see pp. 78–79*). Do the exercise in either a lying-down or a sitting position for 20 to 30 minutes, 2 or 3 times a day.

❋ **Self-massage:** This facilitates circulation in and around the liver. Lie on your back and rub the area from your lower right chest to your upper right abdomen with your right palm from 100 to 200 times. Count each up-and-down stroke as one time. If you get tired, change hands. Do this massage once in the early morning and again just before going to bed. Always rub your hands together to make them warm before starting.

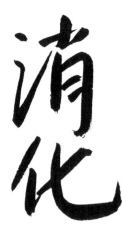

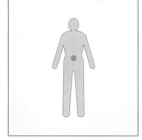

25

ZHEN DUAN HE CHU LI JU LIE WEI BU TONG CHU

Diagnosing and Treating Acute Abdominal Pain

Although acute abdominal pain is a common problem, it is often hard to pinpoint the cause. It can be triggered by functional disturbances in the organs of the abdomen, as well as by defective organs—either inside or outside the abdomen. Sudden spasmodic pains in the abdomen are frequently set off by stomach and intestinal cramping. Persistent abdominal pains may be the result of inflammation. Either inflammation or spasm can cause occasional sharp pains. If the pain comes from cramping, it can frequently be relieved by rubbing and pressing the spot that hurts.

When the pains are confined to a certain area, they may indicate an inflammation. If they are accompanied by involuntary muscular tension, it may signal inflammation of the peritoneum—the membrane that lines the abdominal cavity and surrounds the organs. This is a life-threatening condition and immediate surgery may be needed.

Fixing the site of the pain can provide valuable diagnostic information. If the pain originates in the middle of the upper abdomen, stomach ailments may be to blame. If it is in the right upper abdomen, liver or gall bladder diseases are suggested, although angina (heart pain) and even heart attacks may cause pain in the upper abdomen. A frequent cause of pain in the lower right-hand corner of the abdomen is appendicitis; pain originating in the lower left-hand corner may suggest dysentery, especially when accompanied by diarrhea and blood and pus in the stools. In a woman, lower abdominal pain may also be caused by gynecological or menstrual problems.

Generally speaking, the two best ways of treating acute abdominal pain are through massage or drugs. If you opt for massage, you may find that massaging an acupuncture point far away from the abdomen is the most effective method. It also has the added benefit of not having any of the side effects frequently associated with drugs, and often stops spasmodic stomach and intestinal pain faster than many drugs. After massage, if the pain persists, you should immediately consult your doctor.

Foot-Greater Yang-Bladder Meridian

Have someone massage the acupuncture points on your Foot-Greater Yang-Bladder Meridian, located on both sides of the thoracic vertebrae. A combination of pushing, rubbing, lifting, and holding motions should be used. As you lie on your stomach, the person doing the massage should press with the tip and upper portion of the thumb against the selected acupuncture points. Rhythmical rubbing and pushing against the points with the thumb in a circular motion are best. The speed should be 40 to 60 pulses per minute, and pressure should be applied gradually.

If pain persists, the lifting and holding method can be used: lifting and holding the points with all five fingers 3 to 5 times each. The amount of pressure is about right when you first feel a sore sensation. This massage is good for indigestion.

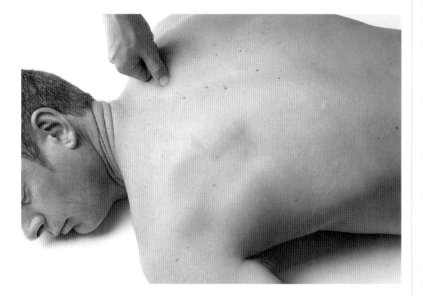

The Foot-Greater Yang-Bladder points are found on either side of the thoracic vertebrae.

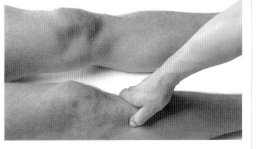

The Tsu San Li point.

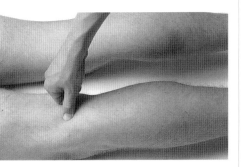

The Wei Chuan point.

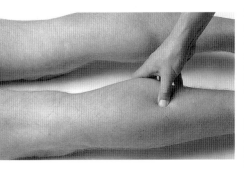

The Shun San point.

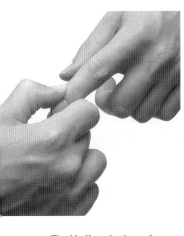

The Ha Ku point is on the index finger, just beside the first joint.

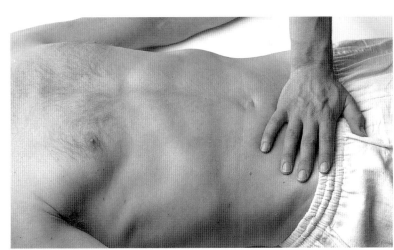

Three acupuncture points

Pinch and knead the three acupuncture points of Tsu San Li, Wei Chuan, and Shun San with a rotating motion, or ask someone to do this for you. Press each point at brief intervals with the tip of your thumb. The pressure should be increased gradually and never applied abruptly. Continue the massage until the point feels quite sore and numb.

If greater pressure seems desirable, use a fast-moving, vibrating motion. Pressing and kneading the Tsu San Li point as hard and deeply as possible is an effective painkiller. If Tsu San Li is chosen as the site for the massage and if you can get someone else to do the massage, you should lie on your back. When Wei Chuan and Shun San are used, however, you should rest on your stomach. Massaging any of the three points is good for relieving indigestion.

Ha Ku and Tan Tien acupuncture points

Ask someone to massage Ha Ku—which is located at the first joint below the tip of the index finger—and Tan Tien—the point 3in (7.5cm) below your navel. Self-massage is not as effective as massage performed by another person. This is good for general abdominal pain.

If you suffer abdominal pain during exercise, you should immediately reduce the level of exercise intensity. Breathe deeply a few times and press and squeeze the painful spot. After this treatment, the pain will usually ease up or even stop. If it does not, you can usually get rid of the pain simply by stopping the exercise.

Tan Tien (the Field of the Elixir), located just below the navel, is used for various abdominal complaints.

Healing Exercises for the Intestine and Colon

There are many possible causes of inflammation of the digestive system: bacterial and viral infection, food poisoning, a long-term poor diet—even stress can be a contributory aggravating factor. However, attention to diet and the positive use of healing exercise can both play a major role in the healing of inflammatory conditions of the intestine and colon.

Although chronic enteritis, which is an inflammation of the intestine, can occur alone, it is frequently accompanied by chronic inflammation of the colon or of the stomach. The most obvious symptom of enteritis is chronic diarrhea, which occurs most frequently during the early morning or after eating a meal.

When enteritis is accompanied by colitis—an inflammation of the colon—constipation, diarrhea, pain in the colon, and the passing of pus, mucus, blood, and undigested foods in the stools may occur. The degree of severity of chronic enteritis and chronic colitis varies considerably. If untreated, the diseases may last from a few years to 30 or more and cause gradual deterioration of the whole body.

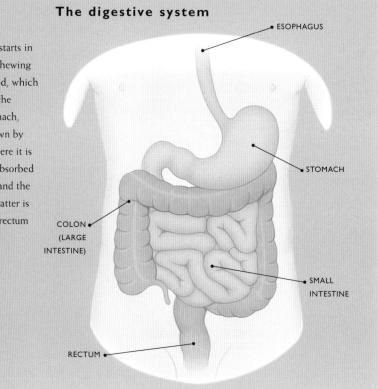

The digestive system

The digestive system starts in the mouth, with the chewing and swallowing of food, which is then pushed along the esophagus to the stomach, where it is broken down by gastric juices. From there it is further digested and absorbed in the small intestine and the colon, before waste matter is excreted through the rectum and anus.

ESOPHAGUS

STOMACH

COLON (LARGE INTESTINE)

SMALL INTESTINE

RECTUM

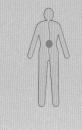

The body's inability to absorb adequate protein, vitamins, and other nutrients due to impairment of digestion can affect the nervous system as well as the metabolism of foodstuffs. Both, in turn, may aggravate the disease. Healing exercise can help the body absorb nutrients, can strengthen organs, and can help regulate the functioning of the nervous system. These benefits contribute to resistance to disease. To work well, therapeutic exercise should be combined with medicine and performed only before the disease has reached a critical stage.

To recover from chronic enteritis and colitis, you need to have faith in the value of exercise and practice it regularly. In the beginning, you can try Fang Sung Kung (*see pp. 72-73*), in the lying-down position. Practice this exercise for 20 to 30 minutes at a time, 2 or 3 times a day. After performing this exercise, massage your abdomen with your palms and pinch and rub your stomach with your thumbs.

When you are recovering, you can practice Tai Chi (*see pp. 60–67*) in addition to other types of exercises. To get the most therapeutic benefit, you should do these exercises 2 or 3 times a day for at least 20 minutes per session.

OBESITY

There are two types of obesity: the kind arising from external factors (exogenous) and the kind caused internally (endogenous). Exogenous obesity is the result of overeating coupled with a lack of physical activity. Endogenous obesity—which accounts for only 3 percent of all cases—is brought about by deficiency in the functioning of the pituitary, thyroid, and other glands. Therapeutic exercise can have only a small beneficial effect in such cases.

By contrast, healing exercise can be extremely effective in treating exogenous obesity, which is by far the most common form of obesity. Do not expect your weight to fall through exercise alone, though.

■ Overindulgence is by far the most common cause of obesity.

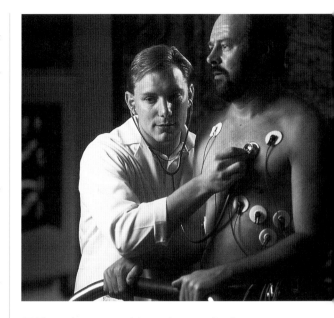

■ Those who are overweight may have associated heart problems, which should be carefully monitored by a health professional.

You must follow a careful calorie-controlled diet at the same time.

There is evidence that the obese have a tendency to store carbohydrates as fat (rather than convert them into the more readily burned glycogen, a body sugar). With less glycogen available to be burned to provide energy, the overweight are more likely to feel hungry and overeat again. In addition, they become less and less likely to exercise because of the breathing and other problems that they experience when they try. If you become aware of a steady increase in your weight, you should act to bring it under control as soon as possible.

A careful and conscientious healing exercise program for treating the overweight can not only reduce fat but can also help treat associated problems such as constipation, hemorrhoids, bloating, and weak heart and lungs. The series of exercises on the following pages (*see pp. 170–173*) have been recommended by Chinese doctors; they are best performed in the early morning. If they are in good health, obese patients may also jog, swim, and play ball games.

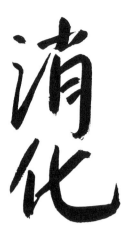

26

NEI CHUANG KUNG

Internal-Strength Exercises

Building up internal strength necessitates increasing the amount of *chi* in the body and having a positive mental attitude, to stimulate the immune system and aid resistance to disease.

1 With the backs of your hands facing each other, bend forward as far as you can without pain. As you bend, say "Huh!" and exhale completely.

2 Stand with your arms at your sides and clench each hand into a fist. Raise your hands as if you were lifting a heavy object with the tops of your fists. Turn your fists so that your fingers face up as your hands reach chest level, and inhale deeply.

ESSENTIAL POINTS

Combine the movements with the correct breathing technique and a positive mental attitude, for optimum results.

SET A

Stand with your feet shoulder-width apart, your toes turned very slightly inward, and your arms at your sides. With the backs of your hands facing your thighs, lift your arms gracefully with your elbows bent, turning your palms until, when they reach chest level, they face up. As you do this, breathe in deeply.

3 Standing with your fists at your sides, fingers facing forward, lift your arms straight out to the sides as you exhale.

1

2

3

4 **While holding your arms out to the side, inhale. Then exhale** as you rotate the backs of your fists forward with your thumbs toward the floor.

5 **Still standing with your arms out, inhale again, and then** exhale as you turn your fists until your fingers are on top.

6 **Inhale and bring your arms down. Press your fists hard** against your abdomen to aid your deep exhalation.

7 **Relax your hands and let your arms hang naturally. Breathe** in and out 3 times before repeating the whole set. Depending on your level of fitness, you can repeat this 10 to 30 times.

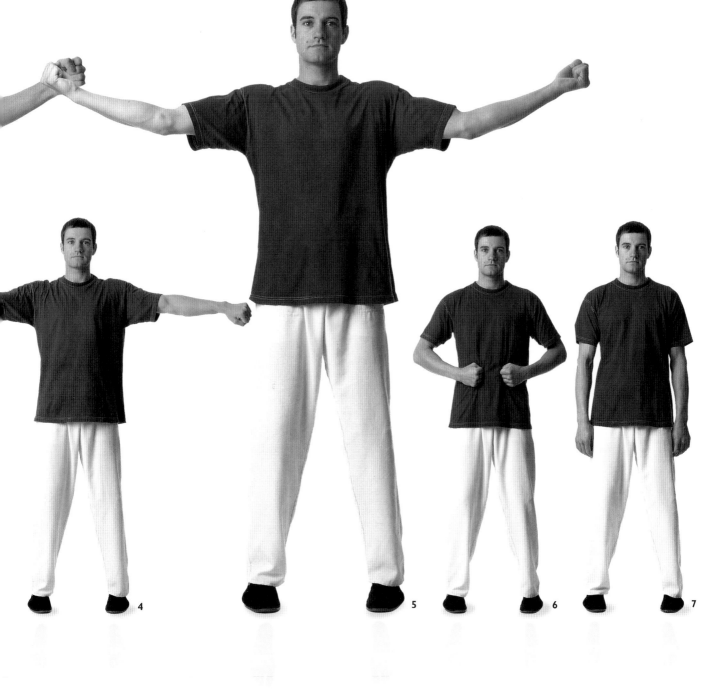

4   5   6   7

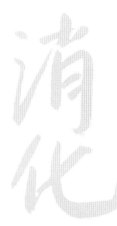

SET B

Position your feet as if you were taking a long step, left foot forward with the knee slightly bent. The distance between the heel of the front foot and the toes of the back foot should be about 24in (60cm). The space defined by your insteps should not exceed 18in (46cm). The toes of your front foot should face forward but those of the back foot should turn slightly out. Keep both feet in place during this exercise, with your weight divided between them.

ESSENTIAL POINTS

■ When done correctly, in a smooth synchronized way, this exercise feels like swimming in the air.

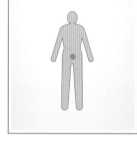

1 **With your feet positioned,** turn your body slightly to the right and let your eyes follow the movement. Bring your hands up in front of your chest with the backs facing each other and your fingers pointing up.

2 **Let your arms swoop gracefully downward.** Then stretch your left hand out in front of you as you extend your right arm back.

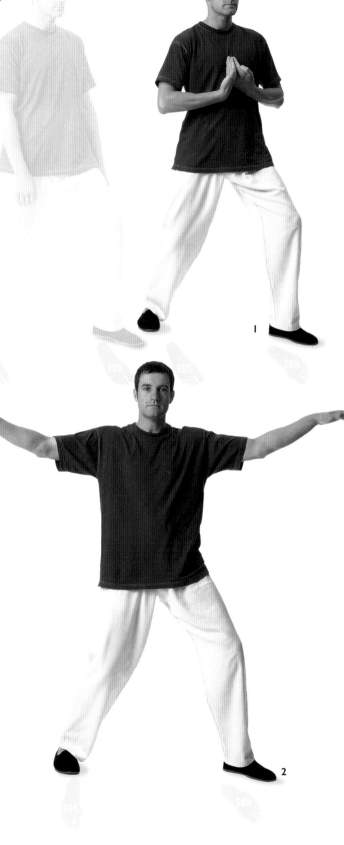

3 Turn your body slowly forward. Then put your right foot forward and follow the instructions in step I, but turning the opposite way. So turn your body slowly to the left, keeping your eyes level as they follow the turn, and bring the backs of your hands together in front of you.

4 Repeat the same moves as in step 2, but put your right arm forward and your left one back. Repeat first to the right, then to the left. Work up to 100 alternating repetitions.

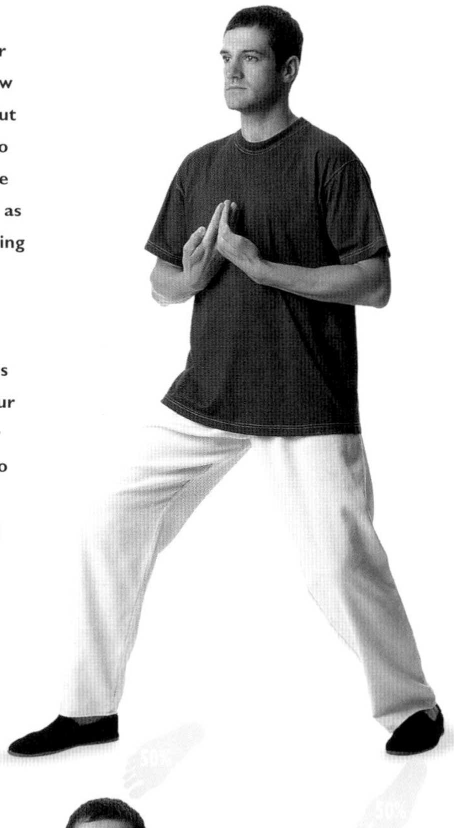

3

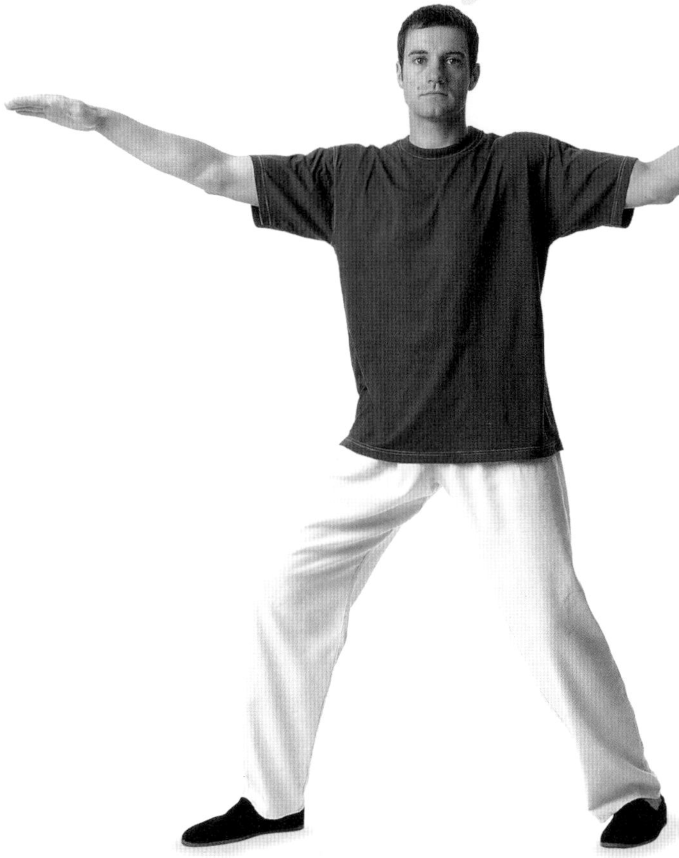

SET C

Stand naturally with your feet parallel to each other about shoulder-width apart. Breathe deeply through your nose for 1 to 2 minutes.

I Do deep knee bends. As you squat, exhale fully, pressing both hands against your abdomen.

2 Inhale as you rise. Repeat 10 to 20 times. Afterward, take a leisurely walk for 10 to 20 minutes.

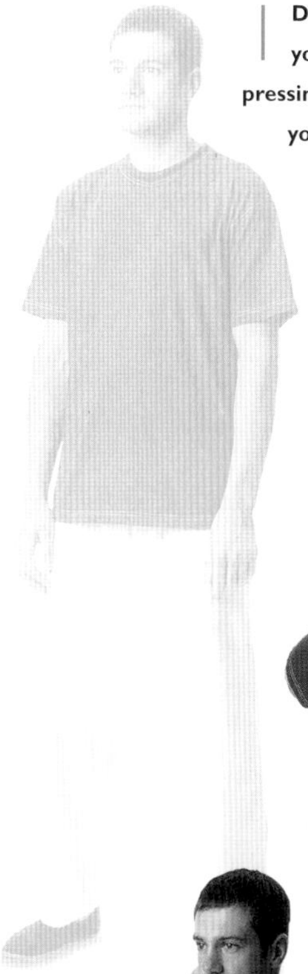

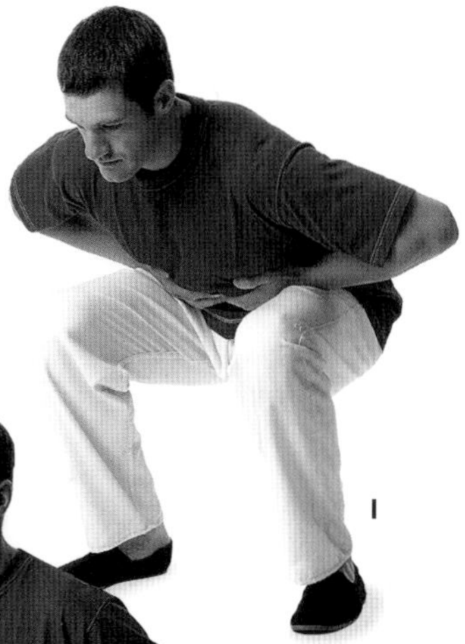

1

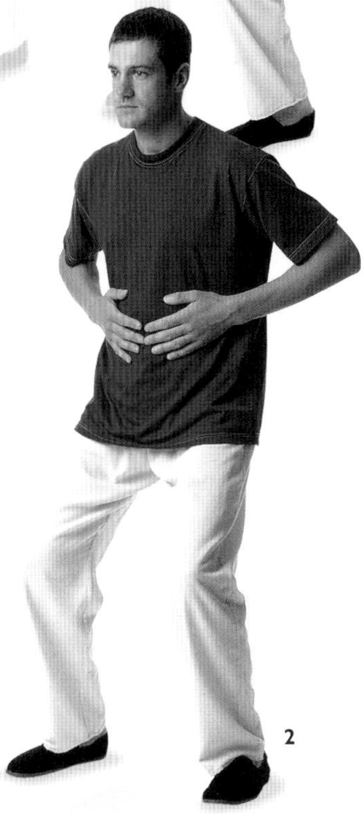

4

2

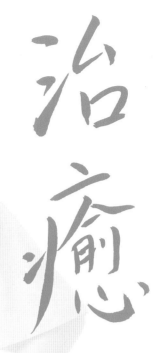

CHAPTER SIX

Healing the nervous system to create a healthy body and mind

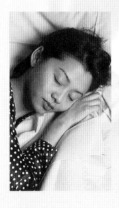

■ **Sleep helps the body and mind to regenerate during the night.**

The nervous system connects the brain and the body, in both directions. If you want your body to do something, a signal from the brain along the nervous system will get you to perform the action. And if you get a cut on your body, the nervous system sends a message to the brain to let it know that an injury has occurred. But for the body/brain to communicate effectively, the nervous system must be healthy and neither over- nor underactive. An excessive intake of stimulants, such as tea, coffee, and alcohol, will make the nervous system overactive, while a diet lacking the essential nutrients will make it deficient.

Illnesses that affect the nervous system produce a wider range of symptoms than afflictions in any other system of the body. From the moping disinterest in life, poor appetite, and insomnia that characterize those who are depressed to an actual inability to walk, nervous-system disorders have unpleasant impacts on our lives, but may be helped by eating a sensible, nutritious diet and following a healing exercise routine.

■ **Depression is increasingly common, due to the stresses and pressures of modern life.**

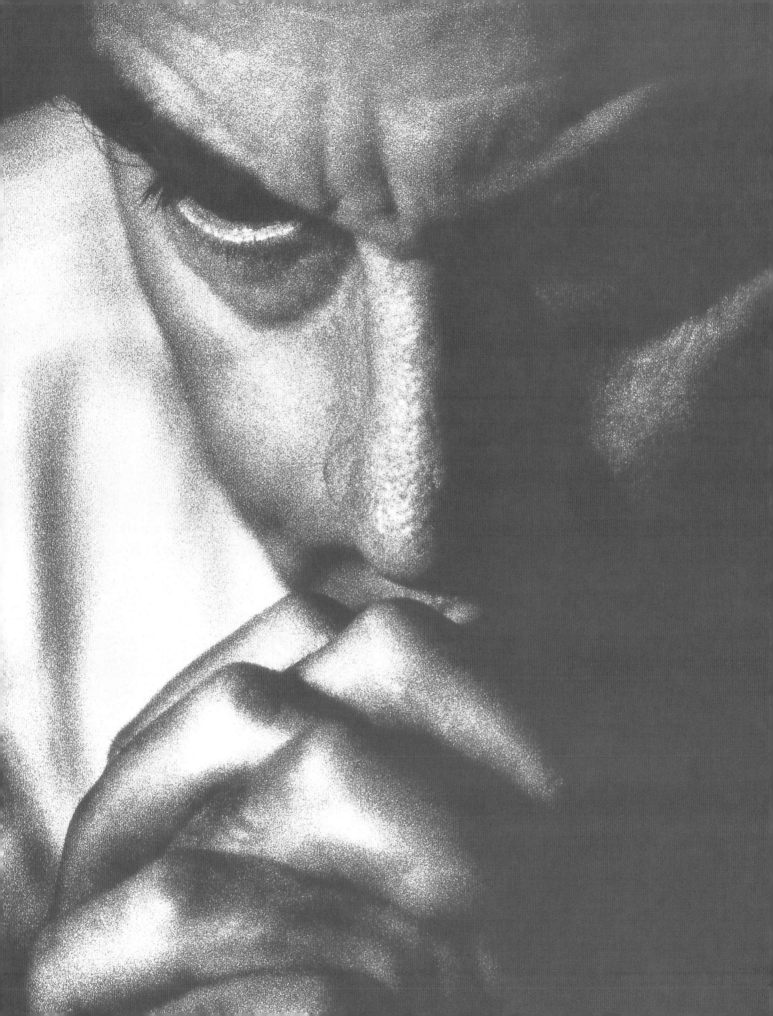

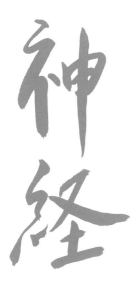

27

DUI KANG QING XU DI LA

Combating Depression

Should depression be treated with rest or exercise? If the depression is caused by exhaustion, rest, and sleep are the keys to revitalizing nerve cells in the thinking parts of the brain. But rest alone is not enough—it is also important for those who are depressed to improve their physical fitness, which will enhance their ability to cope with both home and work situations.

During a workout, muscles and joints feed a steady stream of nerve impulses to the central nervous system, and these transmissions, according to medical professionals, have a regulating effect on the nervous system. Apart from conditioning the nervous system, physical activity also helps to divert the attention of depressives away from an obsessive involvement with their own problems. This helps improve their emotional state and, therefore, also reduces other symptoms.

Rest, exercise, and recreation are all important in the treatment of depression. The effectiveness of exercise varies from person to person because of the individual nature of the problem. Those who suffer from chronic tiredness due to mental strain, overwork, and physical inactivity will benefit the most from healing exercise. If depression is a result of other diseases, treatment should begin by curing the underlying disease before attempting to relieve the depression.

The best healing exercises for treating depression are Tai Chi, Chi Kung, massage, leisurely walking, hikes, and expeditions. Of these, Tai Chi appears to be the most effective.

Tai Chi

In recent years the Chinese have used Tai Chi widely and successfully in treating depression. This exercise offers special benefits because it calls for mental and emotional tranquility. It requires full concentration so that what the mind imagines, the body becomes. Because of its mental and spiritual demands, Tai Chi conditions the nervous system and helps induce feelings of calm and peace. After a reasonable period of practice, Tai Chi will often be able to cure mental distraction and irritability.

Although Tai Chi is rather complicated to learn and it takes time to become proficient, it is well worth the effort. The best way to learn is to take lessons, but you can also follow the technique step by step, as described on pages 62–67. As you study and practice, keep in mind the three key words that describe the movements of Tai Chi: calm, loose, slow.

Chi Kung

In traditional Chinese medicine, Chi Kung is noted for its effectiveness in treating diseases characterized by the qualities known as emptiness, weariness, deficiency, and injury. Chi Kung nourishes *yuen chi*—vital energy—and builds up inner strength. It works on depression mainly because it produces mental quietness. In this state, the exerciser switches off cortical activity—active thinking, worrying, and fretting—and weary nerve cells are given a chance to revitalize.

Chiang Chuang Kung, invigorating breathing (*see pp. 74–77*), is recommended for treating depression. The physically weak may adopt the lying-down position and the physically fit may perform the exercise either standing or sitting. Those who are both physically and mentally weak should try Fang Sung Kung, relaxation breathing (*see pp. 72–73*). You can practice Chi Kung for 30-minute sessions, 2 to 3 times a day.

Massage

Often depression is accompanied by other symptoms, and self-massage can be effective in helping alleviate some of them.

For insomnia and anxiety-related palpitations, rubbing the acupuncture point Yung Chuan

---

ESSENTIAL POINTS

■ To keep the mind and emotions in better balance, you need first to get the body balanced.

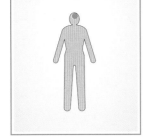

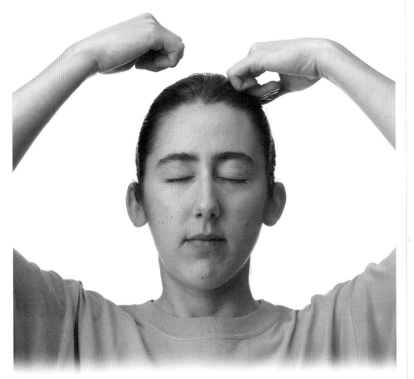

For dizziness, gently tap your head all over; also snap both your index and middle fingers against it while you cover your ears with your palms (see pp. 56–57, set 4).

CAUTION

If you ever experience excessive perspiration, overexcitement, or insomnia, you should reduce the amount of exercise you are doing.

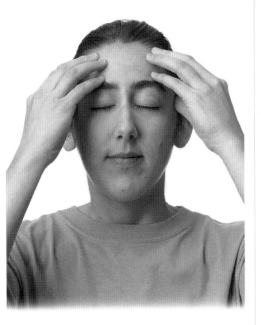

For a headache, rub your face with the same kind of brisk motion you use when brushing your teeth. You can also try massaging the acupuncture points around your eyes (see pp. 90–91).

(Bubbling Spring) is an effective remedy (*see p. 59*). This point is located one-third of the way down the foot, in the depression made when the toes are curled under.

Leisurely walking, hikes, and vacations

A leisurely walk for a distance of 1½–2 miles (2.5–3.2km) can help regulate the excitation and inhibition processes of the cerebral cortex, reducing symptoms such as headaches and throbbing pains in the temples. Many patients have noticed that their mood and spirits improved as a result of regularly engaging in exercise. For the physically fit, field trips and excursions also help divert attention away from their problems.

Other exercises

Exercises such as swimming, table tennis, basketball, canoeing, and similar outdoor exercises are good for the depressed. But for healing exercise to be successful, depressed people should remember that physical activity is only one component in a comprehensive treatment program. Depressives also need to resolve the other problems that may be contributing to the neurosis. They should work on maintaining a proper balance between work and relaxation and on developing a spirit of optimism.

The amount of exercise you should do depends on your physical condition. If you're weak, do only Chi Kung and massage. If you're fit, you can do additional exercise for 30 minutes to an hour. The physically strong may exercise for 1 to 2 hours in both the morning and afternoon.

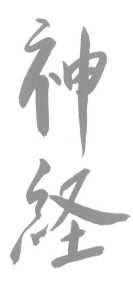

28

ZHI LIAO SHI MIAO

Curing Insomnia

The inability to get to sleep, or insomnia, can be caused by a number of factors, the most common of which are depression and temporary emotional disturbances. For these types of insomnia, sleeping pills are only a temporary cure and in the long term may cause more problems than they solve in the short term. To treat the underlying causes of insomnia, the patient needs to inhibit the overstimulated cerebral cortex and achieve calm. An effective way to accomplish this is through healing exercise.

The following exercises should all be done before you go to bed. You can do them individually or consecutively.

Walking

Take a leisurely walk for 5 to 10 minutes. After you have calmed down, go to bed.

Tai Chi

Perform one set of Tai Chi (*see pp. 62–67*). After you have calmed down, go to bed.

ESSENTIAL POINTS

■ A calm body without tension will enable the mind to be relaxed and quiet.

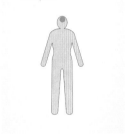

Massage the body all over as if you were taking a dry bath. First rub your face gently with both hands (*see pp. 56–57, set 3*). Then massage your left arm with your right hand, and vice versa. Next, rub the chest and abdominal regions. Your hand movement should be slow and light. Finally, massage the acupuncture point Yung Chuan (*see pp. 58–59, set 11*). Continue massaging until you feel calm and peaceful—usually 10 minutes of self-massage will be enough.

RIGHT HAND RUBS
THE LEFT ARM

Massage

Perform self-massage either sitting down or lying on your back. Cover your body with a blanket if the room temperature is low. You will feel tired and sleepy, so relax your body and go to bed. The type of massage you just gave yourself is valuable because it frequently produces a calming and hypnotic effect.

Fang Sung Kung

You can also do either Fang Sung Kung (*see pp. 72–73*) or Chiang Chuang Kung (*see pp. 74–77*). Or you can simply lie on the right-hand side of your body and let your muscles go loose. Then empty your mind of all thoughts and let it follow the rhythm of your breathing until you fall asleep. Since the purpose of this exercise is to induce sleep, the amount of time spent is not important. Generally, it takes about 10 minutes or so before you feel sleepy.

You can combine these exercises with other techniques, such as soaking your feet in a bowl of warm water just before going to bed. And be sure not to engage in any mental work for 30 minutes before going to sleep. If you wake up after falling asleep, just relax your body and follow the rhythm of your breathing until you drop off again. Above all, try not to worry about the fact that you cannot get to sleep.

Before you go to bed, soak your feet in warm water for 20 or 30 minutes to help relax the body. You can even combine this with the massage technique.

HANDS MASSAGE THE ARMS

FEET SOAK IN WARM WATER

神
経

29

YUN DONG JI LIAO ZUO QU SHEN JING TONG

Treating Sciatica with Exercise

There are many possible causes of sciatica, a nerve condition that usually causes a sharp pain in the buttocks, which radiates into one leg and often into the foot. It is frequently associated with weakness and numbness. A slipped (herniated) disc, osteoarthritis of the spine, and sciatic neuritis (inflammation of the sciatic nerve) can all cause this problem. It is thought that sciatic neuritis may be triggered by the common cold, by absorption of toxins from the environment, or by inflammation of tissues in surrounding areas. It responds well to healing exercise, but you should not exercise during acute attacks; massage and gymnastic exercises can help in the chronic stage.

In the early stages of recovery, after doing the massage below, you can do the exercises that follow.

ESSENTIAL POINTS

■ Acupuncture is another effective treatment for those who are suffering from sciatica.

SET 1 ▌ Massage

For the kind of massage that is most helpful in cases of chronic sciatic neuritis, you will need to prepare a simple but special tool. Wrap or roll a wooden rod in a number of layers of cloth to cushion it. Then tap yourself, starting at the waist and moving around to your back. Do your hips and legs as well. Each muscle group should receive 5 to 10 minutes' attention. Repeat this tapping action 3 to 5 times a day.

SET 2 ▌ Leg straightening

Lie on your back with your feet on the floor and your legs bent. Straighten each leg in turn, keeping your thighs parallel, and hold your leg aloft for 30 seconds.

SET 3 | Knee squeeze

Lie on your back with your feet on the floor and your legs bent. Press your knees together. Then try to separate them with your hands while using your leg muscles to continue to hold your knees against each other. Continue for 30 seconds.

SET 4 | Lying leg swings

Lie on your good side with a slight bend at the hip. Move your affected leg backward and forward gently for a minute or so.

SET 5 | Seated leg extensions

1 **Sit on a chair with your knees bent and lean back on your hands for support. Extend your left leg.**

2 **Bend the left leg, then the right. Repeat 8 times, or fewer if it becomes uncomfortable.**

1

2

After you have improved your condition and are beginning to feel a little better, you can continue with the following exercises.

SET 6 | Shifting weight

With your hands on your hips, put your weight on your right foot, bend your right leg, and extend your left foot to the left side. Then transfer your weight onto your left leg, which should be bent, as your right leg straightens out. Do 8 bends on each side.

WEIGHT IS TRANSFERRED FROM RIGHT LEG TO LEFT

SET 7 | Waist bends

1 **Sit on a chair with your legs slightly bent and place your hands on your thighs.**

2 **Bend forward from the waist and let your hands slide down over your legs to your feet. Repeat 4 times.**

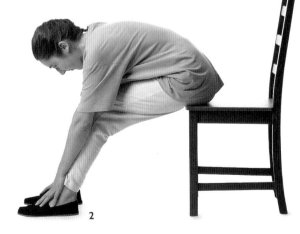

1

2

SPINE BENDS FORWARD FROM THE WAIST

SPINE BENDS BACKWARD

SET 8 ‖ Waist and back bending

1 Stand with your feet shoulder-width apart and your hands on your hips. Lean slightly forward from the waist.

2 Now bend backward from the waist. Repeat 8 times. Gradually increase the distance you bend.

SET 9 ‖ Leg swings

Stand up straight and hold onto something sturdy, such as a chair. Swing your affected leg forward and backward easily. Keep your knee fairly straight, but not locked. Continue for up to 5 minutes.

SET 10 ‖ Toe touching

Sit on a chair with your legs stretched out in front of you. Lean forward gently and try to touch your toes. Repeat several times.

LEG SWINGS FORWARD AND BACKWARD

CHAPTER SEVEN

Relaxing and toning the muscles and bones through healing exercise

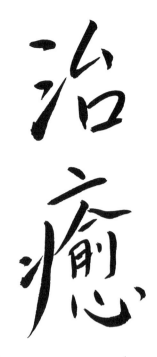

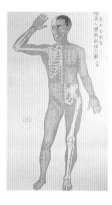

The body's skeleton, muscles and meridians will all be helped by regular Tai Chi.

Making you stronger and more flexible is one gift that healing exercise regularly imparts. As helpful as it is for diseases of the organs and internal systems, its most immediate impact is on the parts of the body involved in movement—the bones, muscles, ligaments, and related tissues.

Such healing exercise can help you reverse the effects of age. Just as nothing makes you feel older than sore, weak, creaking, and painful joints and muscles, nothing contributes more to a youthful feeling than a flexible, strong, and eager body. Even if your body has been bent and misshapen by years of misuse, by lack of use or by disease, healing exercise may be able to help you. The greatest exercise system for overall health and strength is Tai Chi. Practicing this system once a day will help many specific health problems, as well as general fitness and suppleness. All the body's joints, muscles, tendons, ligaments, sinews, organs, nerves, and acupuncture meridians will benefit from its gentle routines.

Exercise can help you retain something of a child's incredible suppleness as you grow older.

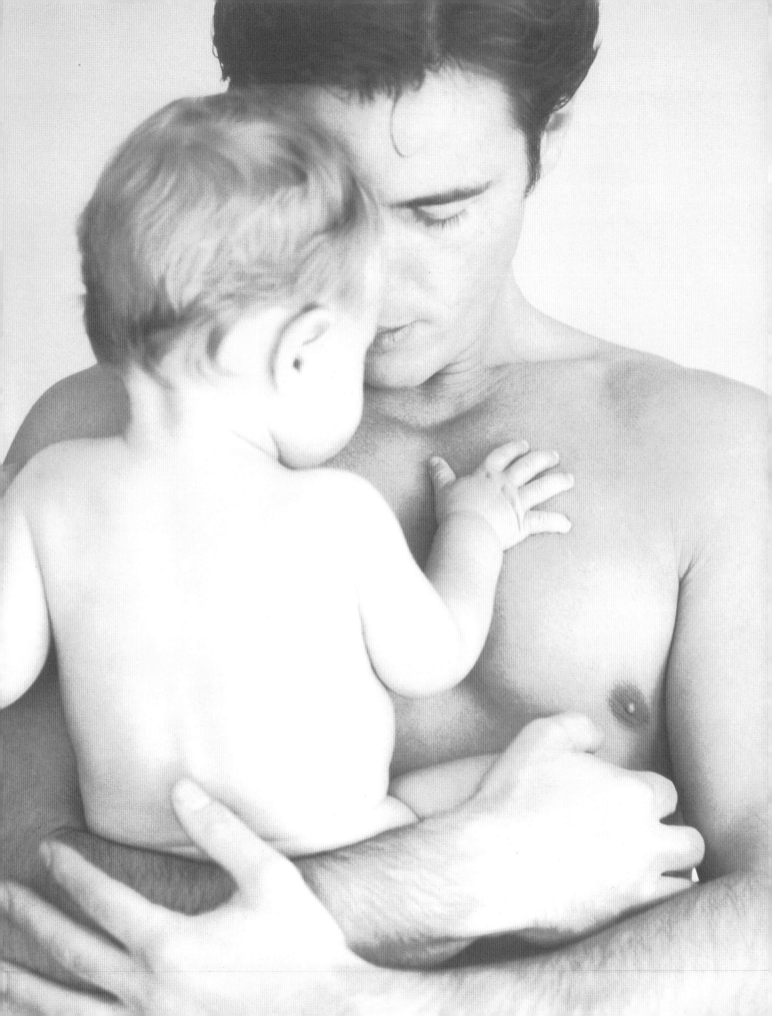

肌肉与骨

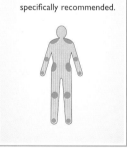
30

YU FANG JI SHU HIAN GUAN JLE YAN

Preventing and Easing Arthritis

The movements of Tai Chi involve every important joint in the body. Regular practice of Tai Chi keeps both bones and joints healthy, making this classic Chinese exercise routine one of the best ways to prevent arthritis. Even those who have already developed arthritis may still be helped by practicing Tai Chi. The exercise's effectiveness will depend on how far the disease has advanced and which joints are affected. You should do Tai Chi only if you can do it without undue pain.

When arthritis is mild, most people will not have extreme pain or stiffness and practicing Tai Chi at this stage will help improve overall health as well as joint mobility. But inflammation in the knees, the small of the back, the sacroiliac joint or other joints that are actively involved in the exercise may serve only to intensify the pain. Patients who have pain in these joints may wish to try out the exercise for a period of time under close medical supervision. If they adapt well and suffer no negative effects, they may continue and expect good results.

Some arthritics do experience pain at the outset, but later find their pain soothed and their overall health improved. However, if your condition seems to be worsening as a result of the exercise, stop exercising—at least temporarily. If you have a significant problem, you may want to consult your doctor about the advantages of exercise for your condition. ›

SET 1 ▌ Stiff fingers

Clutch a pencil or a stick tightly in your fist. Then straighten your fingers and palm by flattening your hand against a table or desk.

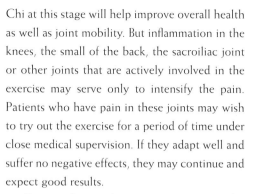

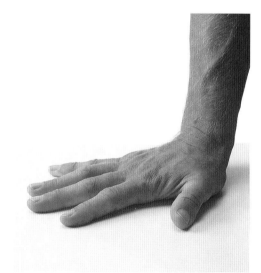

SET 2 ▍ Improving wrist flexibility

Press your palms together in front of your chest. Use each hand in turn to press the other back. Do this rapidly, and don't be afraid to press fairly hard. A light dumb-bell can also be used to build strength and increase mobility in your wrists, as you flex them while holding the dumb-bell.

How exercise can help rheumatoid arthritis

In rheumatoid arthritis the joints are often swollen, painful, and stiff. Healing exercise can help improve joint mobility when the condition is chronic, and it can help stop it from becoming acute. Even when there is acute inflammation, exercise can be of benefit; it can also prevent such flare-ups. The affected joints need exercise several times a day. Exercise rods—an old broomstick will do—can be especially useful in improving flexibility of the joints.

Massage and passive exercise of the affected joints and the surrounding muscles can help ease pain and swelling when other kinds of exercise don't. Rub and knead the joints lightly, but massage your muscles deeply. About the right amount of time to spend on a massage is 10 to 20 minutes. With smaller joints, such as the finger, wrist, elbow, and ankle, start by soaking them in warm water—just about body temperature—for about 10 minutes. This reduces muscle pain and spasm and makes your joints easier to move.

Try any of the exercises on these pages and the next two that are relevant for you. Each exercise may be done 10 to 20 times, preferably at least twice a day.

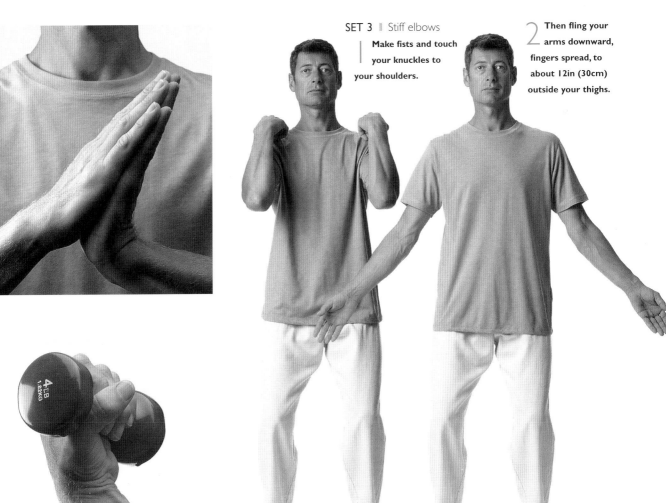

SET 3 ▍ Stiff elbows

1 Make fists and touch your knuckles to your shoulders.

2 Then fling your arms downward, fingers spread, to about 12in (30cm) outside your thighs.

1

2

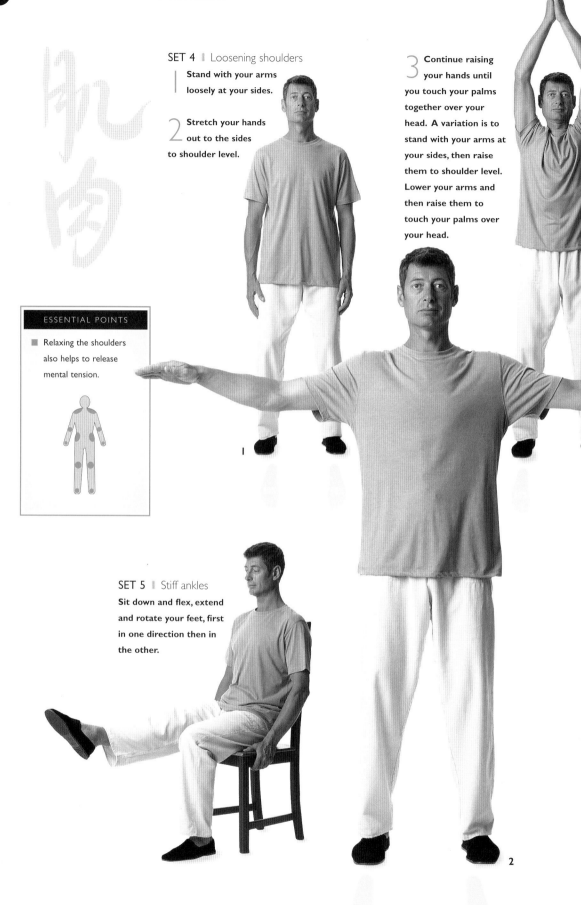

SET 4 | Loosening shoulders

1 **Stand with your arms loosely at your sides.**

2 **Stretch your hands out to the sides to shoulder level.**

3 **Continue raising your hands until you touch your palms together over your head. A variation is to stand with your arms at your sides, then raise them to shoulder level. Lower your arms and then raise them to touch your palms over your head.**

ESSENTIAL POINTS

■ Relaxing the shoulders also helps to release mental tension.

SET 5 | Stiff ankles

Sit down and flex, extend and rotate your feet, first in one direction then in the other.

1

2

3

SET 6 ❚ Curling shoulders

1 ❚ To increase your shoulders' forward and backward mobility, stand up straight and lace your fingers behind your head. Draw your elbows back to open the shoulders wide.

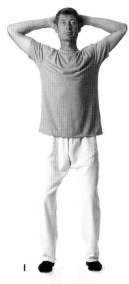

1

SET 7 ❚ Stiff hips and knees

1 ❚ To build flexibility in these joints, take a long step forward and bend your front leg. With your hands on your hips, draw your elbows back and thrust your chest forward. Hold this position until your muscles tire. Alternate legs.

1

2 ❚ Then do deep knee bends while holding onto the back of a chair for support. Keep your heels on the floor.

2

2 ❚ With your fingers laced and the back of your hands against the back of your waist, curl your shoulders forward, as if you were trying to make them meet in front of your body.

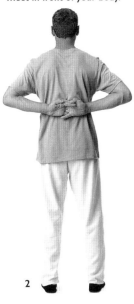

2

SET 8 ❚ Leg swinging

1 ❚ Hold onto the back of a chair, or some other sturdy object, and swing your left leg forward.

2 ❚ Take it back forcefully. Then switch legs and repeat.

1

100%

2

100%

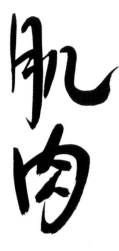

(31)

SHI GE JI CHU SUN SHANG DI YUN DONG

Exercises for Spinal Deterioration

When rheumatoid arthritis acts to fuse the bones of the spine together, the condition is known as ankylosing spondylitis, or Marie Strumpell disease. The spine typically bows out in the thoracic, or chest, region but is flattened in the lumbar region, or middle back. This condition causes stiffness and limits the patient's mobility.

Patients with this disease should do therapeutic exercise to help keep the unaffected joints mobile before the spine becomes completely fused.

If, however, the spine has already completely fused, therapeutic exercises will not be effective.

The exercises should focus on training the muscles of the abdomen, shoulders and hips, since improving these muscles can partially compensate for the inadequate function of the spine. Since this disease limits chest movement, patients are likely to have weak breathing. Therefore, exercises that encourage abdominal breathing and expand the chest region are particularly useful.

Before doing any of the exercises below, lie on your back and do some abdominal deep breathing, as described for Chiang Chuang Kung (*see pp. 76–77*).

ESSENTIAL POINTS

Maintaining spinal flexibility is absolutely essential in order to achieve good health.

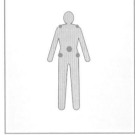

● *Each of these exercises may be repeated 10 times or more, as often as twice a day.*

SET 1 ❙ Feet raising

1 Lie on your back with your hands behind your head. Bend your legs at the knees and draw them toward your abdomen.

2 Then raise your feet up with some force. Relax and lower them.

SET 2 ❙ Flying

1 Lie on your stomach with your arms extended to the sides.

2 Lift your arms up over your back, as if flying.

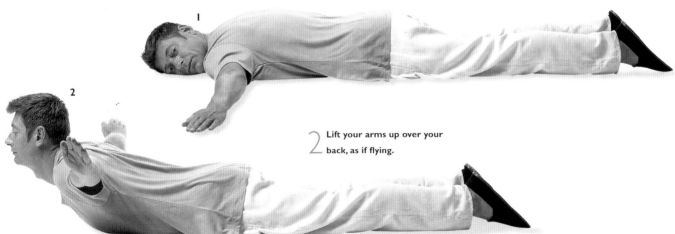

SET 3 | Head turning

1 **Stand with your feet shoulder-width apart and your hands resting on your hips.**

2 **Bend your head forward and backward, then turn it from side to side.**

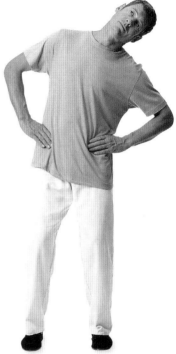

1

2a

2b

SET 4 | Leaning to the sides

Stand with your feet shoulder-width apart and your hands on your hips. Lean your body gently to the right, then to the left.

SET 5 | Sitting with momentum

1 **Lie on your back on the floor and stretch out with your arms over your head.**

2 **Use the momentum of bringing your arms forward to help you raise yourself to a sitting position.**

1

2

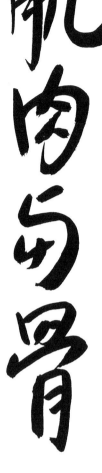

32

ZHI LIAO JIAN GUAN JIE YAN

Healing Arthritis of the Shoulder

Many people over 40 years old, particularly those with chronic diseases, are bothered by painful and stiff shoulder joints. The shoulder joints often feel as if they are glued together and may feel tender while they are being examined. X-rays may also show that both the tendons and bursae (the pads that are supposed to prevent friction) are undergoing calcification. Known as tendinitis or bursitis, this condition causes inflammation in the tissues around joints. Physical exercise can frequently help relieve arthritic shoulders, as well as helping to prevent the type of bursitis that is caused by metabolic problems and general physical weakness from ever occurring in the first place.

Perform these exercises at least once—and preferably twice—every day.

SET 1 ▌ Shoulder rotation

1 **With your arms hanging loosely at your sides, rotate your shoulders so that your** hands make circles beside your body with your shoulders.

2 **Do one shoulder at a time, moving forward for 20 circles and then backward for 20.**

SET 2 ▌ Hand pushing

1 **Put the back of your hand against the front of the shoulder on the same side of the body.**

2 **Push your hand forward as if you were pushing something away from you. Do this** with each arm 10 to 20 times.

ESSENTIAL POINTS

■ The benefits of such exercise are cumulative. It is better to do 5 minutes every day than a half-hour once a week.

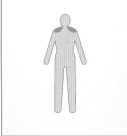

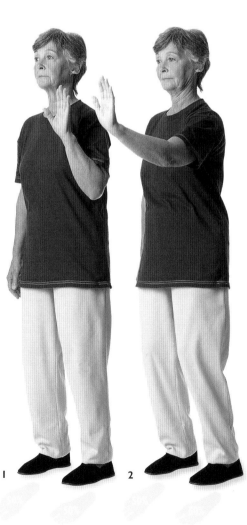

1   2

SET 3 ❚ Hand lowering

1 **Lace your fingers together and stretch your hands high over your head.**

2 **Lower them behind your head. Do this 10 to 20 times.**

FINGERS ARE INTERLACED
ABOVE THE HEAD

SET 4 ❚ Arm swinging

Swing your arms, one forward and one back, like pendulums. Swing vigorously and rhythmically 10 to 20 times.

HANDS ARE LOWERED
BEHIND THE HEAD

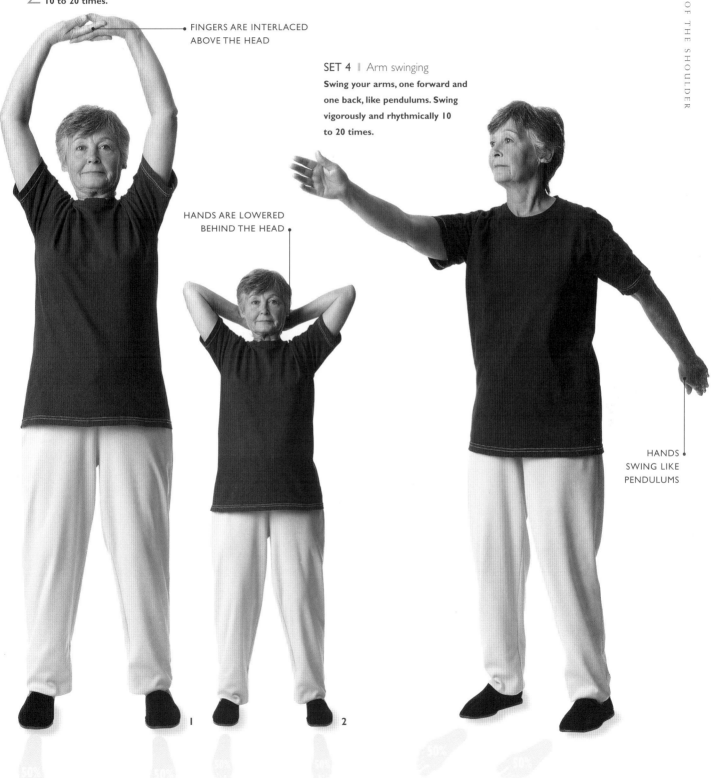

HANDS
SWING LIKE
PENDULUMS

肌
肉

33

SHU HUAN LIAN GUAN JIE TONG

Freeing Frozen Shoulder

Advanced bursitis of the shoulder can cause so much stiffness and so limit mobility that the patient may feel as if the joint has been frozen. In fact, the condition is sometimes called frozen shoulder. If the bursitis is caused by an external injury, physiotherapy should be used with relaxation exercises. If the condition is due to chronic strain—inflammation of a muscle due to overuse of the upper arm—massage, physiotherapy, and the appropriate healing exercises are suitable. But if the condition has been brought on by physical weakness, exercise is the first recourse. Physiotherapy and massage should be used, too. Acupuncture is another successful treatment.

You can select part of the following sequence or do the whole set, depending on your strength and flexibility.

SET 1 | Forward arm raising

1 **Stand in a relaxed position, holding** an exercise rod in both hands in front of you.

2 **Forcefully raise your arms straight out in** front of you and over your head. Lower them again. **Repeat 10 to 20 times.**

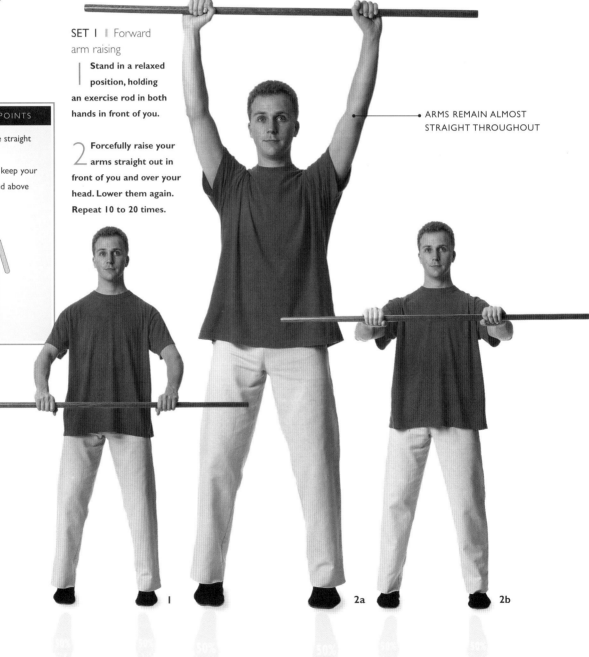

ARMS REMAIN ALMOST STRAIGHT THROUGHOUT

1

2a

2b

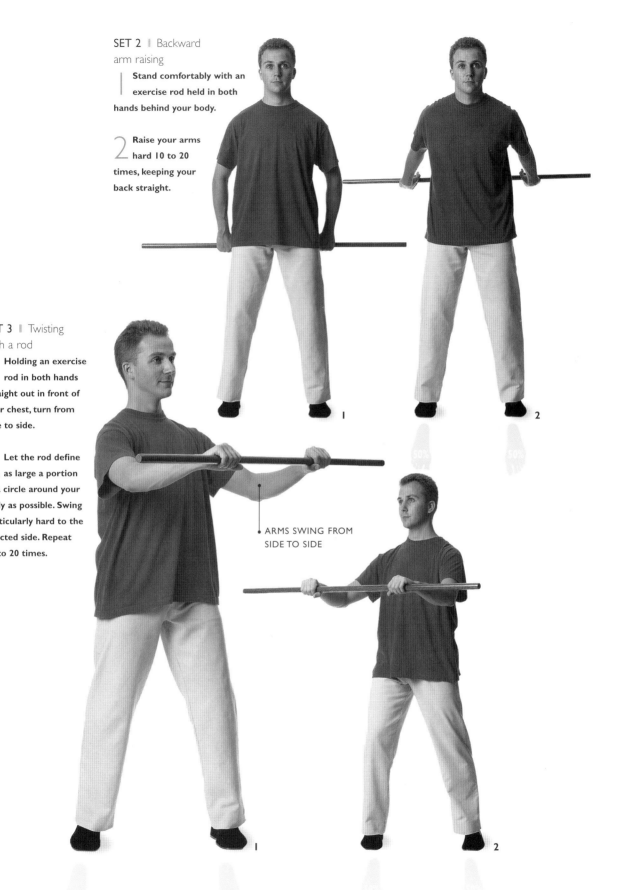

SET 2 ▮ Backward arm raising

1 **Stand comfortably with an exercise rod held in both hands behind your body.**

2 **Raise your arms hard 10 to 20 times, keeping your back straight.**

SET 3 ▮ Twisting with a rod

1 **Holding an exercise rod in both hands straight out in front of your chest, turn from side to side.**

2 **Let the rod define as large a portion of a circle around your body as possible. Swing particularly hard to the affected side. Repeat 10 to 20 times.**

ARMS SWING FROM SIDE TO SIDE

SET 4 ❚ Elbow raising

Stand with your feet shoulder-width apart. Raise the elbow of the affected arm as high as you can and touch the back of your neck with your hand, without bending your back. Repeat 10 times.

HAND REACHES TO BACK OF NECK

SET 5 ❚ Spinal reach

Stand with your feet shoulder-width apart and your back straight. Reach behind your waist and raise your hand as far up your spine as possible. Alternate with your other hand and repeat at least 10 times.

SET 6 ❚ Elbow reach

| Stand with your feet shoulder-width apart and your back straight. Lace your fingers together behind your neck.

2 Turn your elbows as far to the back as possible, as if you were trying to touch them together. Repeat 10 times.

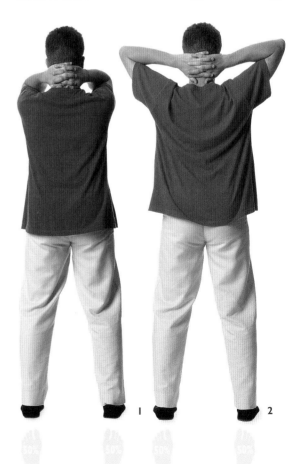

ESSENTIAL POINTS

■ Try to keep the spine straight and vertical.

■ Relax the body as much as possible.

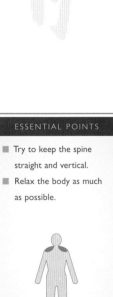

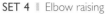

1

2

SET 7 | Hand raising behind

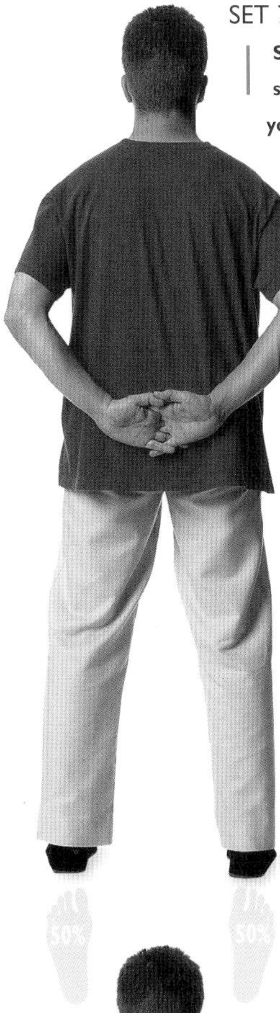

Stand with your feet shoulder-width apart and your back straight. Lace your fingers together and place your hands, palms facing out, against the back of your waist.

2 Raise your hands as high up your back as possible before returning them to your waist. Repeat 10 times without bending your body.

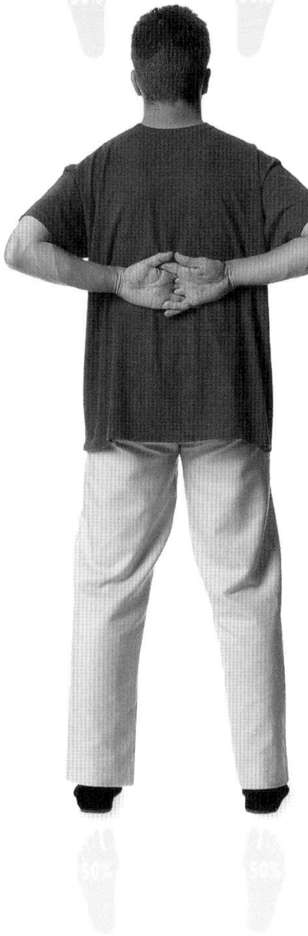

1

2

SET 8 | Reach for the sky

Stand with your back straight about 12in (30cm) away from a wall, ladder, or tree. Place the hand of the affected arm on the object at about shoulder level. Gradually move your hand higher.

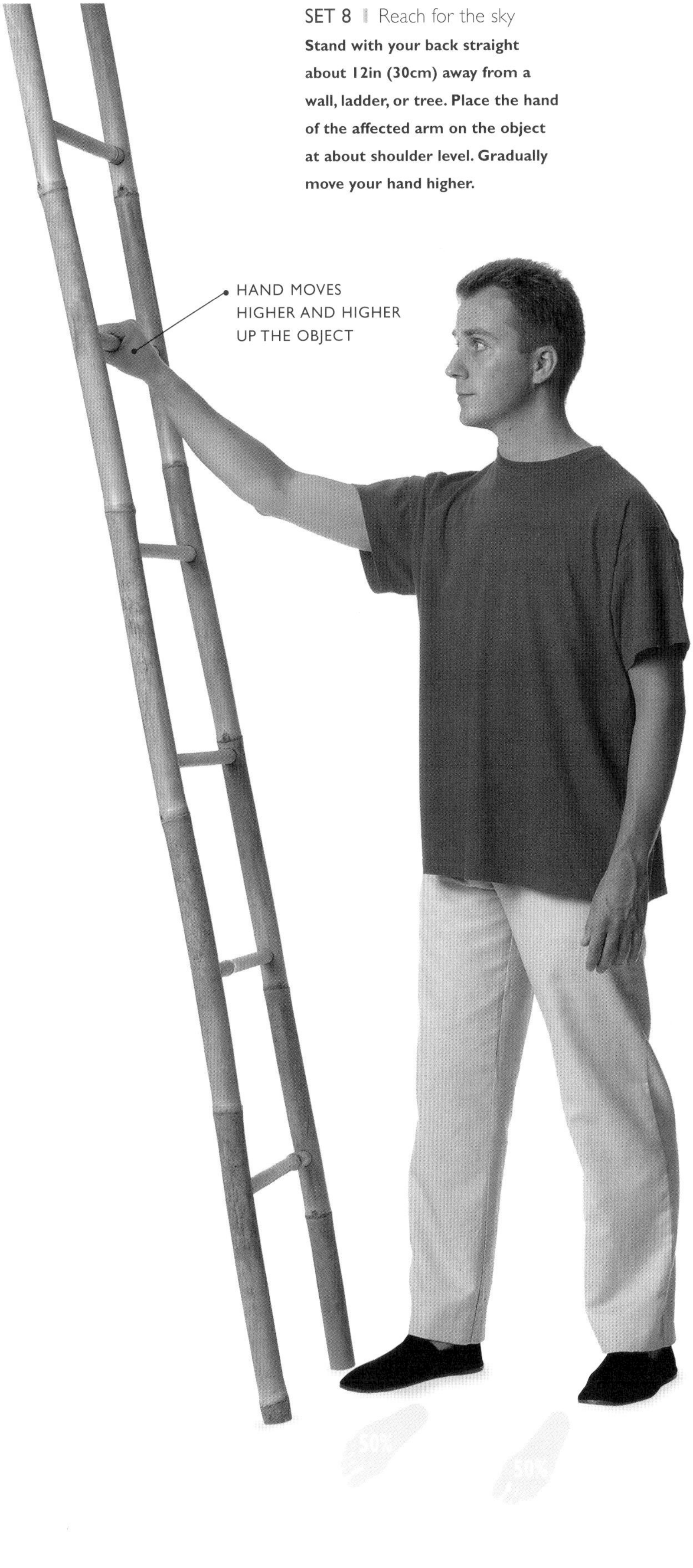

HAND MOVES
HIGHER AND HIGHER
UP THE OBJECT

肌肉与骨

(34)

SHU HUAN XIA BEI TONG ZHI YUN DONG

Exercises for Lower Back Pain

Lumbago, or pain in the lower back, is only a symptom, not an actual disease in itself. The causes of lumbago can be quite varied. One of the most common types—functional lumbago —is mainly a result of incorrect posture or weak muscles of the back and the loin. Posture-induced lumbago is brought about by an exaggerated forward curve in the lumbar region of the spine. When a person has this forward curve, the stress on the vertebrae may cause inflammation and may result in pain.

Another type of functional lumbago, found more frequently in the elderly or the physically

SET 1 ▌ 90-degree leg raises

1 **Lie on your back and lift your legs to an angle of about 90 degrees, keeping the small of your back pressed to the ground.**

2 **Move your legs slightly to your left side and lower them slowly.**

3 **Raise them again, but this time move them slightly to the right and lower them. Repeat 3 to 4 times.**

1

2

3

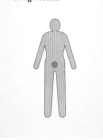

inactive, is caused by weak muscles of the back and loin. Both abdominal and back muscles lack the strength and resilience to support the lumbar vertebrae in bearing the weight of the body. People with this condition who have to sit, stand, or walk in the same position for a prolonged period often get backache. Carrying heavy objects or bending their back is difficult for these people. Their weak muscles force the ligaments and joints of the lumbar vertebrae to carry too

great a share of the burden. As a result, painful lumbago develops. Exercise, if it is done correctly, helps prevent lumbago because it encourages proper posture and strengthens the muscles in the abdomen, loin and back. Strong muscles in these areas and correct posture are essential to support the spine. Persons who frequently bend their back in the course of heavy work or strenuous exercise should do preventative exercises even if their back muscles are well developed.

SET 2 ‖ Scissors kicks

1 Lie on your back and lift your legs about 45 degrees, keeping the small of your back presse to the ground.

2 Do scissors kicks in the air until your muscles become tired. Rest for a minute, then repea the sequence 3 to 4 times.

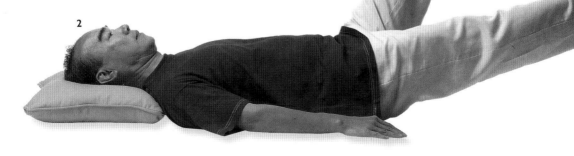

SET 3 ┃ Back arching

1 | Lie on your stomach with your elbows bent, your upper arms in a straight line with your shoulders, and your hands in front of your head.

2 Raise your upper body and your arms and legs off the floor and hold this posture for a moment. Repeat several times.

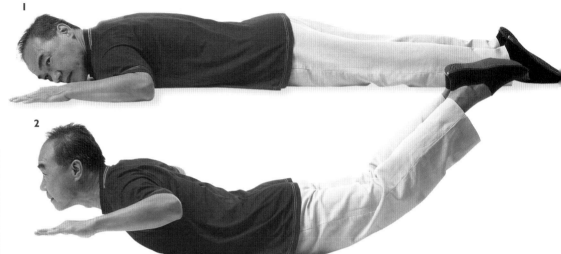

ESSENTIAL POINTS

■ Over-exertion of the back muscles is not beneficial.

■ Feel the effort, but don't do it to excess.

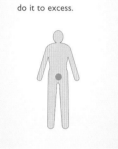

SET 4 ┃ Partial sit-ups

1 | Lie on your back with your hands resting on your hips, your legs straight out in front of you and your head on a cushion.

2 Raise your head and shoulders off the floor in a partial sit-up. Hold for as long as is comfortable— your abdominal muscles should be doing the work— then return to the start position. Repeat several times.

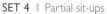

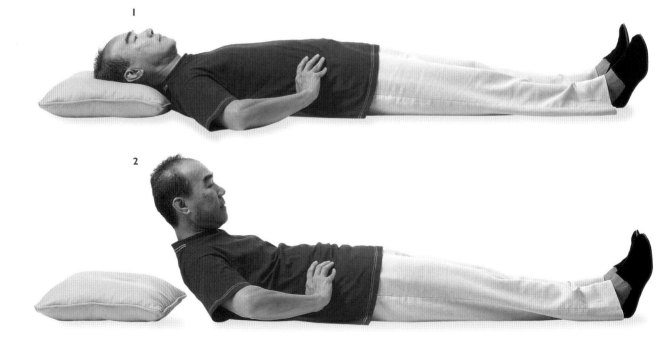

SET 5 ▌ Body bow

1 **Lie on your stomach on the floor, clasp your hands and place them in the small of your back.**

2 **Draw your body into the shape of a bow by lifting both your upper body and your legs.**

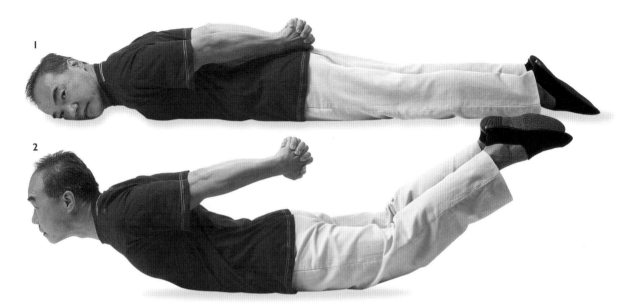

SET 6 ▌ Alternate leg raises

1 **Lie on your stomach on the floor, with your hands palm-down on the floor by your sides.**

2 **Lift your legs alternately. Repeat several times.**

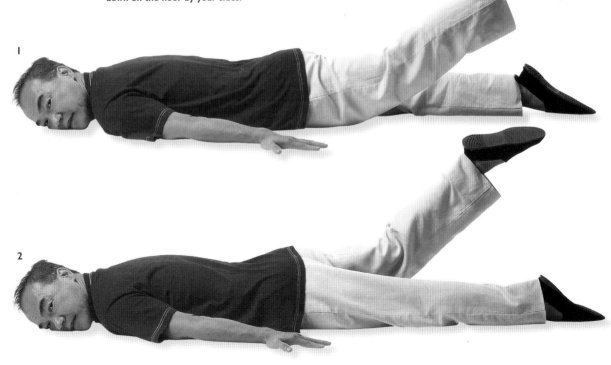

35

YUN DONG ZHI LIAO YAO TONG

Healing Loin Strains with Exercise

When the loin muscles—the muscles located in the sides between the pelvis and ribs—are injured, the sacrospinalis muscle, which extends the vertebral column, is usually involved, too. Muscle injury may result from a sprain or a pull. If untreated, the resulting bleeding and leaking of other fluids can put pressure on nerve endings, causing pain, as well as making fibrous tissue form. The fibrous tissue itself can trigger pain during muscle contractions.

Exercises designed for treating this condition focus primarily on relaxing the muscles of the loin and the lower back and increasing mobility in the spine. Exercises that involve tensing the muscles of the loin should be avoided. You can perform all the exercises, or select just a few. Repeat each exercise 10 times.

ESSENTIAL POINTS

■ Focus on the part of the body that is being specifically worked in each exercise.

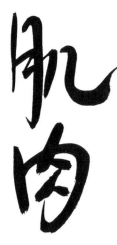

SET 1 | Leg lifting

1 **Lie on your back with your arms at your sides. Lift one leg at a time.**

2 **Raise each leg as close to 90 degrees as you can get it. Your movements should be quick but unstressed, and they should not cause pain.**

1

2

SET 2 ‖ Knee hugging

Lie on your back, bend your knees and draw your legs toward your abdomen. Hold your knees with both hands to press your back firmly against the floor. Keep the loin and the lower back muscles relaxed.

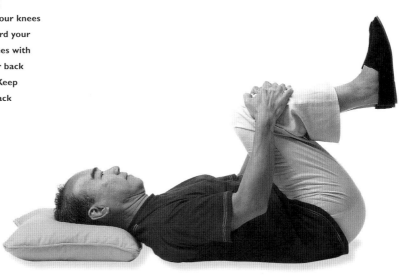

SET 3 ‖ Sit-ups

1 Lie on your back on the floor, with your arms by your side and your head on a cushion.

2 Use your abdominals to raise you into a sitting position. You can lean on your hands for support if necessary. Do not bend your body past a 90-degree angle with your legs.

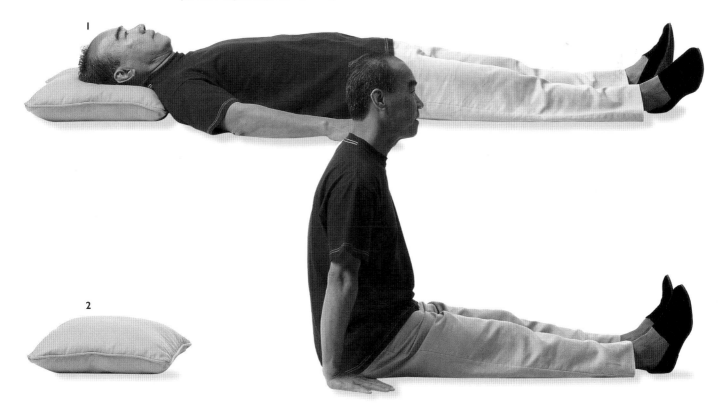

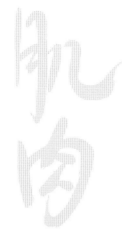

SET 4 ▎ Arm flinging

1 **Stand with your hands on your hips and turn your body** quickly to the left. As you turn, fling your left arm out and up in the direction you are turning and let your eyes follow your outstretched palm.

2 **Let your hand circle around and return to your hip as you** turn in the opposite direction and stretch out the other arm.

LEFT ARM IS
OUTSTRETCHED

EYES FOLLOW THE
RIGHT ARM AS IT IS
OUTSTRETCHED

ESSENTIAL POINTS

■ Try to keep the spine straight and vertical.

■ Keep the nose directly over the navel, so that the head moves with the body.

● *If you perform each of these exercises 10 times and repeat the whole set at least 4 times a day, you should note marked relief in no more than a month.*

1

2

SET 5 | Splitting wood

Stand with your feet wide apart and clasp your hands together.

SET 6 | Lunges

Perform a slow, lunging step with your front leg bent and your back leg straight. Hold for a few seconds. Switch legs.

SET 7 | Twisting

Stand with your feet apart and place your hands in the small of your back. Feel the motion in that area as you twist first to the left and then to the right.

1

2 **Lean forward as though you are splitting wood, following the action all the way through your legs. Your motion should be easy, loose, and should not cause pain.**

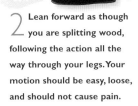

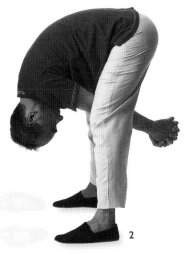

2

SET 8 | Massage

Massage your back and waist area, concentrating on the small of the back, the abdomen and sides (*see pp. 208–209, self-massage*).

1

2

肌
肉
与
骨

36

GAI SHAN XI GUAN JIE

Preventing Knee Strain

Knee strain is a common problem. In its early stages you may feel a weakness and fragility in the knee joint even though you can still engage in physical activity. But whenever you extend your leg, relax it and then push the kneecap downward, you feel pain. If you treat the problem at this stage, it can be improved relatively easily.

Most people, however, do not seek treatment until the condition has worsened and the joint has become swollen. As this deterioration occurs, you usually feel a painful soreness below the kneecap, but the symptoms may fluctuate from mild to extremely painful, depending on activity, temperature, and other factors. At this stage, if you press your hand against the kneecap and move it around, the friction will be audible and the sensation painful. Pain may also be triggered merely by contracting the quadriceps muscle of the thigh, the muscle most important in straightening the leg and most closely connected to the kneecap. If the condition is serious and of long duration, the quadriceps muscle may even have atrophied through disuse.

SET 1 ▍ Backward squat

1 Stand about 18in (46cm) away from a wall with your feet shoulder-width apart. Lean your back against the wall and squat down until your shins and thighs form a 90-degree angle. Let your shoulders relax and hang naturally. Try to maintain this position until your muscles tingle.

2 When your strength has grown, you can move your feet closer to the wall so that the angle at your knees is approximately 80 degrees. In this position, lift your buttocks away from the wall slightly without lifting your heels off the ground. After 1 to 4 minutes in this position you should feel warmth in your quadriceps muscle in both legs. Stop the exercise when your quadriceps begin to tremble and it hurts too much to continue. Walk around for a little while and then repeat the squat 2 or 3 times.

ESSENTIAL POINTS

■ Prevention of knee strain is better than cure.

■ Daily practice will bring results.

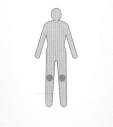

1

2

Some people have shied away from exercise or other physical activities because they feared that it might aggravate the pain or worsen their condition. But this can in fact compound the problem because lack of physical activity inevitably leads to shrinkage of the leg muscles, which in turn affects joint stability and tissue metabolism, making them prone to further injury. Exercise, if done properly, can improve the blood supply to the muscles and regenerative and connective tissues surrounding the kneecap. As a result, there is an improvement in the metabolic process in the cartilage, bone, and muscle.

Healing exercises for knee strain

As long as you avoid friction between the kneecap and the femur—that is, do not bend your knee at an angle between 105 and 150 degrees—any exercises designed to strengthen the muscles and ligaments in the knee joint are beneficial. Gentle exercise of the quadriceps muscle assists in stabilizing the condition. The combination of exercise and deep breathing also can help lessen pain. Massage can improve muscle elasticity and help prevent shrinkage. The forceful knocking technique (*see pp. 208–209, massage, step 2*) is best done during or toward the end of the exercise.

SET 2 ‖ Horse-riding posture

1 Stand up straight with your feet parallel to each other—the distance between them should be about 3 times the length of your foot. Grasp the ground firmly with your toes.

2 Squat down halfway so that your thighs and shins form a right angle. Make your hands into tight fists and hold them, fingers up, in front of your waist.

3 Standing up straight, breathe in and out deeply and slowly. Do this exercise for a few minutes at first, but extend the time gradually as your kneee condition permits.

ESSENTIALS OF PREVENTING KNEE STRAIN

◆ Warm up properly before exercising, paying particular attention to the quadriceps muscle in the thighs.

◆ Follow an orderly training program suited to your age, skill, and strength.

◆ If one knee is injured, take care that the other does not overcompensate and become injured itself.

◆ Try to avoid running on a too-hard field, as this can put excessive pressure on the knee joints.

◆ Don't stop abruptly after fast running—slow your pace and then walk to a halt.

◆ Keep the knees warm and protected from wind and moisture.

1

2

3

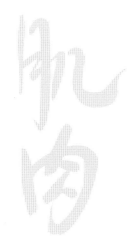

When you have gained sufficient physical strength, you can take the opportunity to do some upper arm exercises while still working on your knees. The deep breathing aspect will help redirect your attention away from any pain.

SET 3 ▌ Fist circling

1 **Still in the horse-riding posture** (*see pp. 206–207*), move your left fist in a semicircle to the left side and up to a position straight over your head while breathing in deeply. Lower your hand through a semicircle to your left thigh while breathing out fully. Breathe in and out several times.

2 **Return your left fist to the original position in front of your waist and lift and lower your right fist in the same manner. Then perform the same exercise with both arms simultaneously.**

ESSENTIAL POINTS

■ Try to keep the spine straight and vertical.

■ Keep the nose directly over the navel.

1a

1b

1c

2a

2b

SET 4 | Palm pushing

1 | In the same horse-riding posture, interlace your fingers, turn your palms away from you and push both your hands out to the front while breathing in and out deeply.

2 Then turn your palms toward you and draw them back near to your chin as you bend forward from the waist in a slight bow, breathing out deeply. Hold this position as you breathe in and out fully several times.

SET 5 | Quadriceps building

Sit on a sturdy stool or chair, lift your legs and hold them off the floor slightly farther apart than your shoulders. Your toes should point up, with your feet at right angles to your legs; your knees should be straight. Hold your arms in front of your chest as if they were wrapped around a large tree. Alternately tense and relax your quadriceps. If you lack the strength for this exercise, you can leave your heels on the ground and use your quadriceps muscle to draw your kneecaps upward.

SET 6 | Self-massage

1 Stand with your feet parallel to each other slightly more than shoulder-width apart. Keeping your legs straight, reach around with both hands and rub and press with a downward motion in the small of the back all the way to the end of your spine. Rub the sides of your hips and bend forward as you massage down the outer sides of your legs and feet. Do not bend your knees or tense your quadriceps muscles.

2 Rub in circles along the outer edges of your feet and toes, and then massage the inner edges of your feet. Massage upward along the sides of your legs until your hands reach your knees. Carefully but repeatedly strike, knock and knead around each knee and the quadriceps muscle on the front of the thigh.

3 As you straighten up, finish massaging the tops of your legs. Work up to your abdomen. When your hands have reached the navel area, continue the massage around your sides until they return to the starting place in the area of the lower back. Repeat the sequence several times and try to relax as much as possible throughout.

1

2

1

2

3

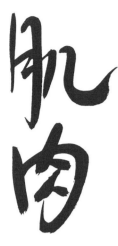

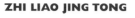

ZHI LIAO JING TONG

Healing Shoulder and Neck Pain

Sometimes, especially in the elderly, the cushioning disks between the vertebrae in the neck protrude, creating pressure on the spinal nerves and triggering symptoms of pain and stiffness in the head, neck, shoulders, and back. The symptoms of so-called cervical disk syndrome may be aggravated by bending or rotating the head.

At times, the pain seems to radiate from the neck to the shoulder and arm, restricting the movement of the cervical vertebrae. Some people's neck movements may have become so restricted their neck muscles have shrunk.

Cervical disk syndrome is treated in the first instance by doctors using pressure-release techniques, such as traction, neck pulling, and massage, and by using drugs and physiotherapy to suppress pain and reduce inflammation and swelling. Therapeutic exercise can be used to help increase the range of motion of the head, neck,

ESSENTIAL POINTS

- Keep the neck and shoulders as relaxed as possible.
- Keep the feet flat on the ground.

SET 1 ▍ Head turning

1 **Sit on a chair with your back straight. Slowly turn your head** to the right.

2 **Keeping your gaze straight ahead, slowly turn all the way** to the left, and then back again to the right.

SET 2 ▍ Pronounced nodding

1 **Sit on a chair with your back straight. Bend your head** forward, with your chin pointing to your chest.

2 **Bend your head backward as far as it will comfortably go** and look up. Don't hunch your shoulders as you do the exercise.

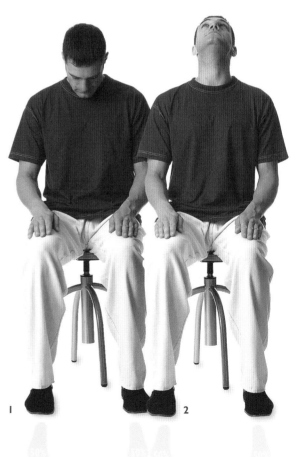

1   2   1   2

and back, as well as strengthening the muscles in these areas. It also improves blood circulation and lessens inflammation.

Healing exercise for cervical disc syndrome consists mainly of head-turning exercises. Your movements should be slow and even, and they should not cause pain. Do not make hard, abrupt moves. When you have reached the maximum stretch, for example at the end of a series of repetitions, hold the position for 1 minute. This will build up muscular strength as well as help lengthen shrunken muscles and ligaments. Start with just 1 to 4 repetitions of each exercise. Work up to more, but stop whenever you feel tired. The first two exercises, head turning and pronounced nodding, are the most important. Work up to doing them for 10 to 15 minutes at a time, 3 or 4 times a day.

SET 3 ▎ Head tilting

1 **Sit on a chair with your back straight. Tilt your head to the right and raise your face toward the ceiling. Feel the stretch from your jaw to your neck.**

2 **Tilt your head to the left and feel the stretch again.**

SET 4 ▎ Head circling

Sit on a chair with your back straight. Let your head roll slowly in a complete circle, then reverse the direction.

SET 5 ▎ Shoulder hunches

1 **Hunch one shoulder toward your ear, and then the other.**

2 **After alternating shoulders for a while, raise both shoulders simultaneously. This exercise is good if the muscles in your neck and shoulders are so tense that it affects the movement of your head. If so, do this exercise before the head circling.**

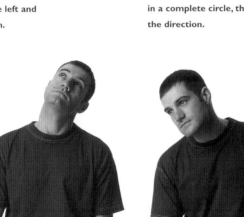

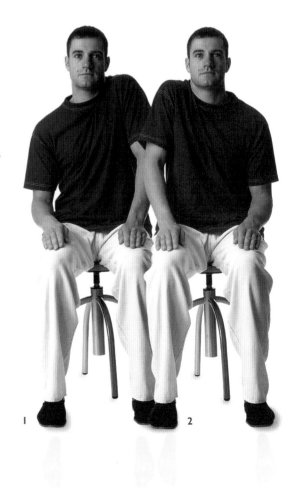

肌肉与骨

38

GAI SHAN JIAN BO

Correcting Rounded Shoulders

Physically inactive people who read, write, or sew in a sitting position for long periods are more inclined than most people to develop rounded shoulders. The nature of their work requires that their arms are continuously in front of their body. As time passes, the major muscle of the chest, the pectoral, shrinks while the major shoulder muscle of the back, the trapezium, becomes slack and weak. As a result, the shoulders turn inward and slant down. To prevent this, people who do this kind of work should make a point of doing exercises designed to expand the chest muscles.

SET 1 ▌ Pushing elbows back

Stand up straight and touch the back of your neck with your finger tips. Draw your elbows as far back as possible. Keep your head high. Hold this position for several minutes before relaxing.

SET 2 ▌ Chest expansion

1 **Touch your hands together, palms facing inward, in front of you at shoulder level.**

2 **Swing your elbows to the rear to expand your chest. Repeat several times.**

ESSENTIAL POINTS

■ Try to keep the spine straight and vertical.
■ Keep the knees slightly bent and loose.

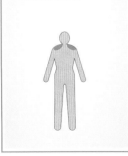

1

2

Some people have protruding shoulder blades, or winglike scapulas, which resemble chickens' or birds' wings. Their problem is caused by weakening of the anterior serratus muscle, which fails to hold the shoulder blades in position. They should try the touching shoulder blades exercise.

SET 3 | Touching shoulder blades

1 Stand comfortably and let your arms hang down naturally by your sides.

2 Lift your hands to a position just above your shoulders, with your palms down and fingers curled.

3 Thrust your chest forward and try to make your shoulder blades touch. Hold for as long as you can. Try to make sure that the movement comes from your chest rather than your waist.

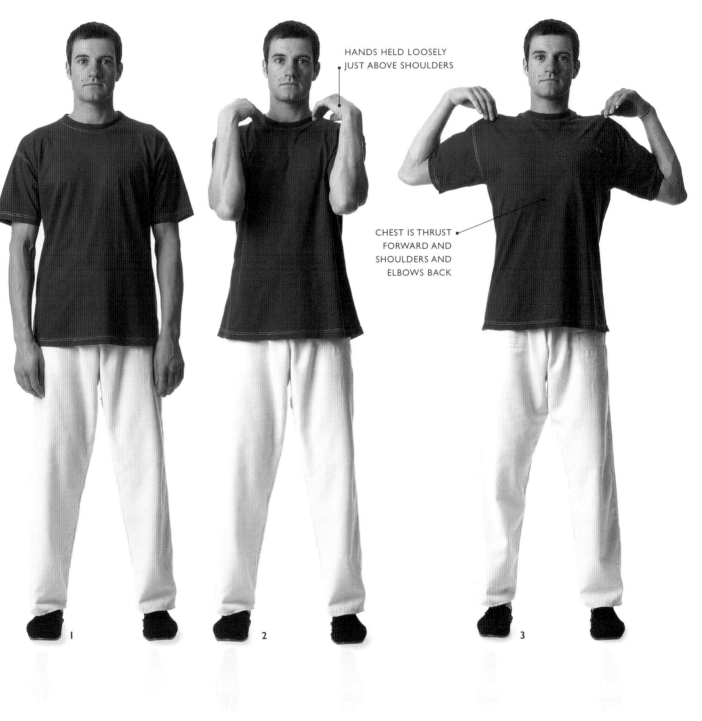

HANDS HELD LOOSELY
JUST ABOVE SHOULDERS

CHEST IS THRUST
FORWARD AND
SHOULDERS AND
ELBOWS BACK

1

2

3

肌
肉
与
骨

39

YUN DONG YU JIE CHUI QU DU

Exercise for Spinal Curvature

Anormal spine goes straight up and down and does not curve to either side. Scoliosis is a condition in which there is spinal curvature. There are two types: sickle- or C-shaped curvature, in which the spine curves only to one side; and snake- or S-shaped curvature, in which the upper and lower sections of the spine curve to opposite sides.

Scoliosis can also be classified by causes. Rachitic scoliosis results from rickets, caused by a deficiency of vitamin D in the diet; underdeveloped bones and muscles, compounded by poor posture and prolonged sitting, are responsible for the damage. Another type results from tilting the pelvis for a long period; the most common causes of this are a misdistribution of body weight to one side while sitting, an

SET 1 ▌ Sideways arm swings
Stand up straight with your right hand resting on your hip. Raise your left arm over your head by swinging it up sideways with force.

SET 2 ▌ Lunges
Stand with your hands on your hips. Take a long step forward with your left leg and bend it. Leave your right leg straight. In this position, stretch your left arm above your head while you reach down forcefully with your right.

SET 3 ▌ Body bends
Kneel with your hands on your hips. Raise your left arm and bend your upper body to the right.

ESSENTIAL POINTS

- Spinal flexibility is essential for good health.
- Exercise only until you feel a little tired.

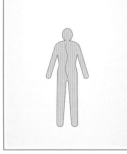

● *Repeat the arm exercises using alternate arms.*

inequality in the length of the legs or one leg being weaker than the other—usually because of polio or other serious illness, so that the pelvis is forced into an unnaturally crooked position. The last type is habitual scoliosis; some children develop lateral curvature of the spine as a result of incorrect reading and writing postures.

Once it is noticed, scoliosis should be treated as early as possible. Corrective exercises are more effective for children and adolescents than for adults, and their success depends on the degree of curvature. Stretching the spine and toning the back muscles form the primary focus, as well as strengthening overstrained and weakened muscles caused by a convex curvature and stretching shrunken muscles caused by a concave curvature. The following exercises can help correct S-shaped curvature. Do each until you feel slightly tired.

SET 4 ▌ Rod twist

Lie on your stomach and hold a long exercise bar (or any wooden bar) with your left hand stretched out in front and your right hand stretched down behind your back. Raise your head and upper body.

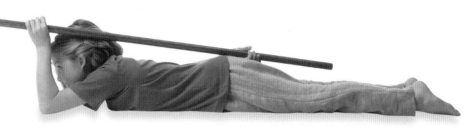

SET 5 ▌ Pillow lying

Lie on the right side of your body with a solid pillow (or sandbag) under the most protruding part of the curvature.

SET 6 ▌ Opposite arm and leg raises

Get down on all fours. With your right palm and left knee on the ground for support, lift your left arm and right leg and extend them. Then do the same on the opposite side.

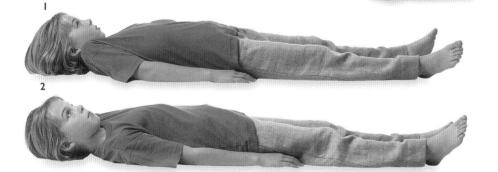

SET 7 ▌ Back creep

1 **Lie on your back with your arms at your sides.**

2 **Inch your way forward, one shoulder at a time, using only your back muscles and shoulder blades.**

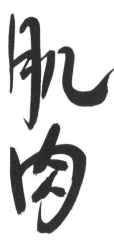

40

MA AN BEI YUN DONG

Exercises for Saddleback

Lordosis—the medical name for hollow back or saddleback—refers to the condition in which the spine has an excessive curve toward the front. It can result from habitual bad posture, from uncorrected post-pregnancy temporary lumbar displacement, or simply from weak back muscles. In children, the condition is frequently caused by a combination of malnutrition and weak muscles, the result of stomach or intestinal disease. These children must be given adequate nutrition as well as corrective exercises.

Except for its unusual appearance, saddleback may not cause other symptoms. In women, however, it frequently causes lumbago, or lower back pain. Exercises designed for correcting saddleback focus on stretching muscles in the lower back and strengthening the abdominal muscles. Do each of the following exercises as many times as feels comfortable.

ESSENTIAL POINTS

■ A straight and vertical spine is highly beneficial in maintaining overall good health.

● *The two bicycling exercises are physically demanding. If you find them too difficult to complete, then you can perform other, simpler exercises designed to strengthen the abdominal muscles, such as those on pp. 150–151.*

SET 1 ▌ Wall touching

1 **Sit on a stool with your back against a wall.**

2 **Pull in your abdomen until your lower back touches the wall. You can also do this exercise sitting on the floor with your legs straight out in front of you.**

LOWER BACK PRESSES FLAT AGAINST WALL

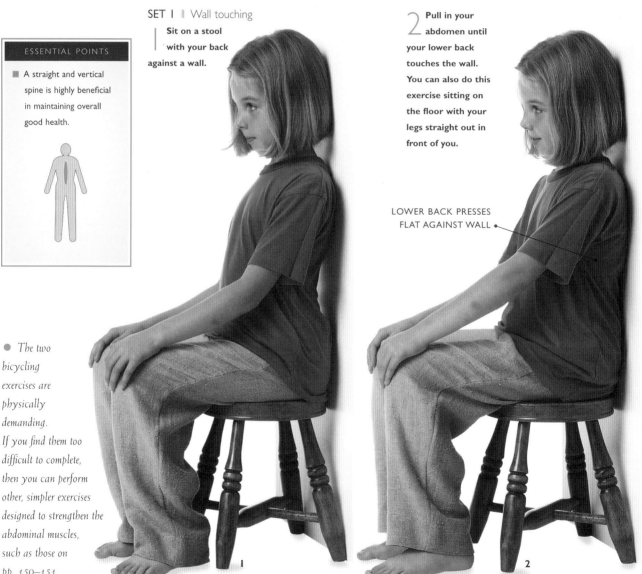

SET 2 ❘ Bicycling behind the head

1 Lie on your back with your knees bent and your palms on the floor. Raise your feet back and over your head. If you wish, you can support your hips with your hands.

2 Bring your legs together and bicycle with your feet by stretching and retracting your legs. The larger the circles that you make, the better.

SET 3 ❘ Upright bicycling

1 Lie on your back with your arms behind your head, then raise your legs so that your hip joints are bent at a 90-degree angle.

2 In this position, bend and stretch your legs one after the other as if riding a bicycle.

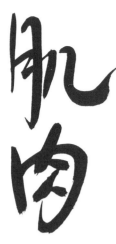

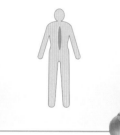

④

YUAN BEI YUN DONG

Exercises for Round Back

Round back refers to the condition in which there is a semicircular protrusion of the upper back. Viewed from the side, a person with round back may be seen to have a protruding upper spine and forward-leaning head and shoulders. When the condition is mild, it does not appear to affect any physiological processes. When it is serious, it can interfere with breathing and cause upper back pain.

There are believed to be three types of round back. The adolescent type, frequently seen in children and teenagers, may be caused by underdeveloped back muscles, using a desk that is too low, inadequate room lighting, and near-sightedness—conditions that force the child to bend

SET 1 ▮ Arm swings

1 Stand with your legs together and extend both arms out in front of you.

2 Swing your arms to the rear as forcefully as you can. Stretch and repeat.

SET 2 ▮ Back arching

1 Stand with your legs together. Keeping your arms straight, lace your fingers behind your back, at buttock level.

2 Stand on tiptoe and raise your arms as you arch your back and thrust your chest forward. Keep your head up.

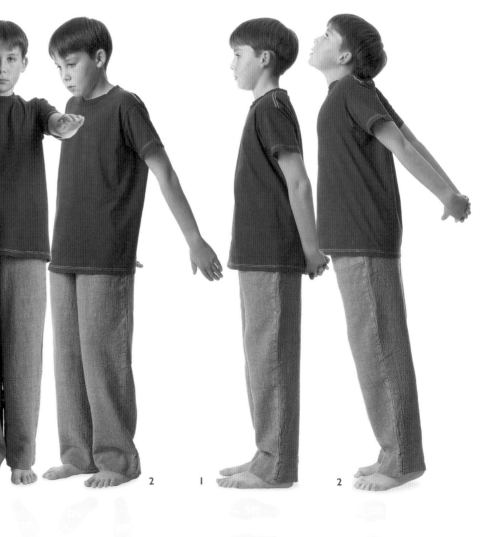

1　　　　　　　2　　　　　　　1　　　　　　　2

SET 3 | Trunk stretching

| Stand with your legs together and hold an exercise bar (or any wooden bar) horizontally in your hands in front of you.

2 Lift your arms with enough force to stretch your trunk.

forward. It may also be hereditary. Occupationally induced round back occurs when a person's job demands too much forward bending. In the elderly, round back may result from an alteration in the tissues of the spinal disks, which in turn weakens the back muscles. The spinal column no longer receives proper support and the thoracic vertebrae curve toward the back.

It is important to prevent the adolescent type by using desks of the right height, providing adequate light in classrooms, and encouraging children to exercise. But round back can be corrected through healing exercises, which strengthen the back muscles, stretch the trunk, and expand the thorax. Repeat the following sequence as many times as you like. Gymnastics and swimming are also helpful.

SET 4 | Body twist

| Stand with your legs together and hold an exercise bar behind your back at shoulder-blade level in both hands, with your fingers facing forward.

2 Turn your body to the left and right as you stretch your trunk.

SET 5 | Squat with exercise rod

| Stand with your feet apart and hold an exercise bar behind your shoulders.

2 Squat halfway down while keeping your back straight.

肌肉与骨

42

JI XIONG ZHENG ZHUANG

Pigeon-Breast Exercise

Some people have a chest that resembles that of a pigeon or chicken. Their breastbone, or sternum, sticks out and the sides of their chest are slightly sunken. Pigeon breast is formed in early childhood. Because of chronic tonsilitis or other obstructions to the airways, some children develop respiratory problems. They cannot take in enough air and their thorax does not expand as it does in healthy children. Their ribs fail to form a natural bend. As time goes by, these children become pigeon-breasted. Young children who suffer from rickets, due to dietary vitamin D deficiency, have underdeveloped bones and are also prone to develop pigeon breast. If the deformity is slight, pigeon breast may rectify itself as the child gets older. If it is serious, the abnormality may become permanent.

ESSENTIAL POINTS

■ You should train to the point of exhilaration, but not exhaustion.

SET 1 ▌ Dumbbell lifts

1 Use dumbbells to strengthen your chest muscles by raising small weights from your sides.

2 Bring your arms up to shoulder level and hold them there for a few seconds. Repeat several times.

DUMBBELLS ARE LIFTED TO SHOULDER LEVEL

SPINE REMAINS STRAIGHT

1

2

Affected children are susceptible to bronchitis and pneumonia because of their weak lungs and inefficient breathing. They should be examined by a doctor. If their problem is related to chronic tonsilitis, therapy should involve clearing the respiratory tract of infection. These children should also be taught to practice deep breathing, with emphasis on proper inhalation. They should breathe in through the nose and out through the mouth. If their condition is caused by rickets, they should be given plenty of vitamin D in nutritional supplements and should be encouraged to exercise somewhere they can get plenty of sunlight and clean air.

Corrective gymnastics and exercises, including running, jumping, swimming, and playing basketball are also recommended. By late adolescence and adulthood, pigeon breast can no longer be corrected. However, individuals with this problem can still strengthen their chest muscles and improve their breathing with the following exercises.

SET 2 | Arm swings

Swing your arms forward and backward, either with or without a dumbbell in your hand.

2 **Hold the arms at shoulder level for a few seconds. Repeat several times.**

1

2

SET 3 | Circling

Make circles beside your body, either with or without dumbbells.

CHAPTER EIGHT

Healing the genitourinary system by means of exercise

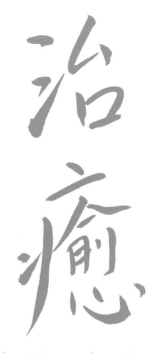

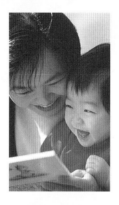

■ **Easier childbirth is just one benefit of healing exercise for the genitourinary system.**

Healthier babies, a fast delivery, and a speedy recovery from childbirth are just a few of the benefits of healing exercises for the genitourinary system. Men with prostatitis and vesiculitis can also be helped. By increasing and regulating energy flow, stimulating the circulation, and building flexibility, strength, and resilience, these exercises can make getting better both easier and faster. And all of these techniques can be used to help prevent painful health problems before they start.

Developing muscle tone through internal exercise of the pelvic and urogenital diaphragms will help to maintain the health of not only the genitourinary system, but all the internal organs in the torso. As human beings—unlike other mammals, which have horizontal spines, with their main organs hanging from them—we have all our organs located on the pelvic and urogenital diaphragms, due to our vertical spines. We therefore need to take this into consideration as part of our daily exercise routine.

■ **Women in particular can gain from healing this system, although men too can benefit.**

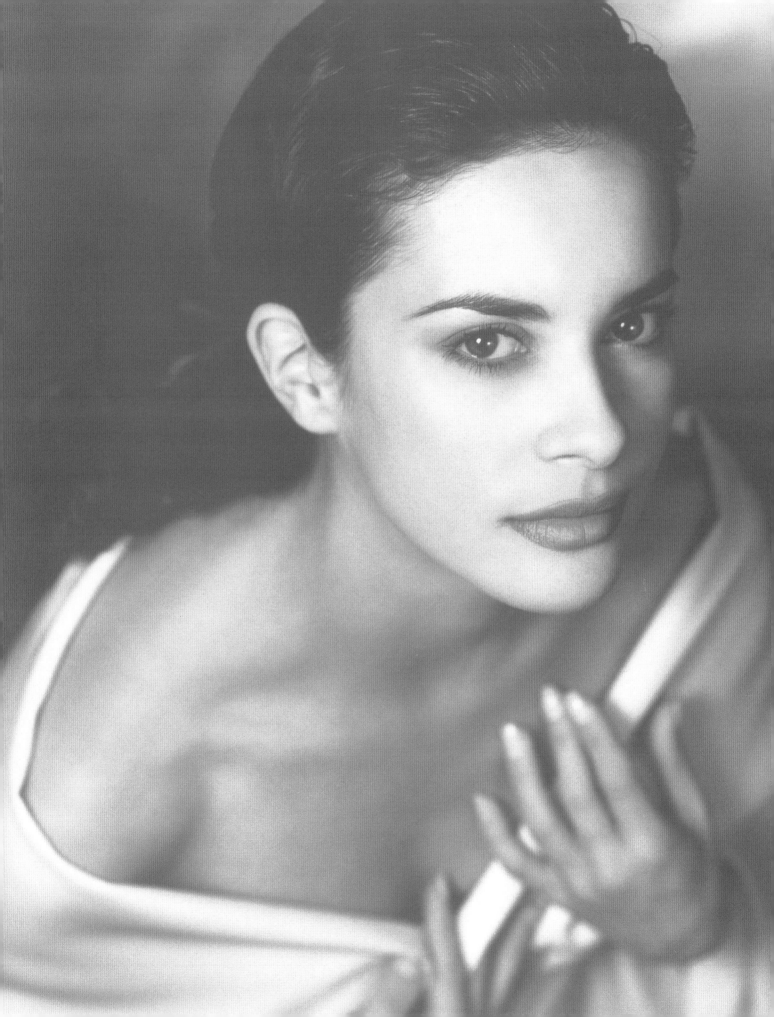

生育

Exercises for Easier Pregnancy and Birth

Continual contraction and relaxation of the pelvic and urogenitary diaphragms, in conjunction with breathing exercises, are extremely beneficial for the general health of both men and women, no matter what their age. In particular, pregnant women will benefit from such exercise, with an easier childbirth and quicker postpartum recovery times.

Pelvic-floor muscles during pregnancy

The pelvic-floor muscles of a pregnant woman are under a great deal of pressure, undergo considerable stretching, and lose much of their tone. Daily exercise will keep them strong and enable them to regain their tone quickly after childbirth has occurred.

MUSCLES OF ABDOMINAL WALL

PELVIC-FLOOR MUSCLES (PARTIALLY HIDDEN BY UTERUS)

Because humans walk on two feet, not four, the soft tissues that make up the pelvic floor have to absorb pressure exerted by the weight of the entire upper body. Upright walking also makes it more difficult for venous blood to return to the heart. In addition, there is a tendency to overlook exercise for this part of the body, especially by women who have sedentary jobs that require them to remain stationary for long periods. As a result, pregnancy and labor may overstrain and weaken the muscles of the pelvic floor and the abdominal wall, causing some of the internal organs to be displaced downward.

During pregnancy, the body undergoes many changes. For one thing, the developing fetus limits the movement of the diaphragm, interfering with respiration. Moreover, there is an increasing demand on the circulatory system. Disturbances in metabolism may also occur.

Therapeutic exercise can strengthen the muscles that support internal organs, as well as improving circulation, helping to keep the heart healthy and reducing chronic inflammation. It can also help improve respiratory functions and speed up the metabolic process. In addition, regular exercise can strengthen the diaphragm and abdominal muscles, making for an easier labor and a smoother delivery. And postpartum recovery time is quicker if pelvic-floor exercises are practiced during pregnancy.

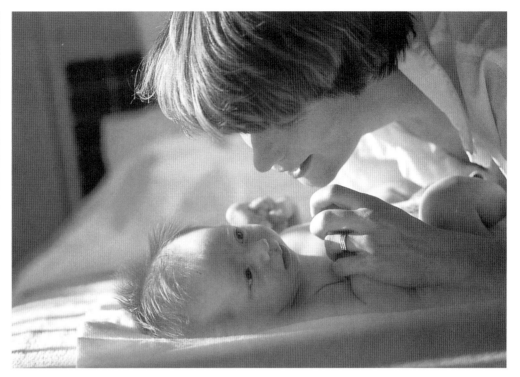

Exercise begun 12 to 16 hours after the birth can help restore physical strength and speed up the tightening of overstretched muscles in the new mother's abdominal cavity and pelvic floor. Clinical studies have shown that, for women who engaged regularly in exercise after giving birth, it took less time for the uterus to contract back to its normal shape and for their urinary and bowel functions to return to normal.

Pregnant women should also exercise to benefit their unborn child. Studies have shown

■ **Both mother and baby can benefit from pelvic-floor exercises undertaken during pregnancy.**

that expectant mothers who are physically inactive—who do not even walk very much, sometimes out of fear—are more likely to give birth to children who are less healthy than the babies of active mothers. Babies of inactive mothers have also been shown to be more likely to develop heart disease. Healthy mothers make healthier babies.

■ **Deep breathing exercises, if done correctly, will help improve body tone and speed up delivery.**

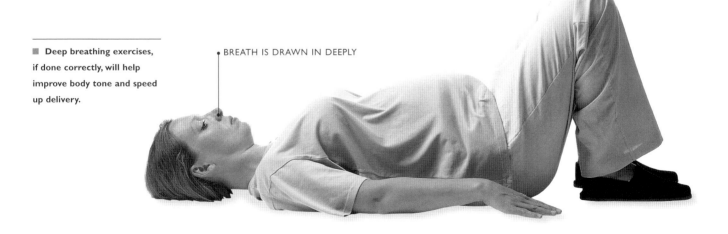

BREATH IS DRAWN IN DEEPLY

生育

43

HUAI YUN JI ZHI YUN DONG

Exercises for Pregnancy

The first trimester of pregnancy is the riskiest for miscarriage because the fertilized egg has not yet firmly implanted itself into the uterine wall. Women who have a history of miscarriage should not exercise during this period.

Most pregnant women, however, will experience no particular problems with occasional short-distance walking or performing deep breathing. Relaxation breathing exercises may help to lessen any problem with morning sickness, which is often characterized by nausea, vomiting, or loss of appetite.

The following set of exercises is recommended for women in the second trimester, between the fourth and sixth months of pregnancy. You can do all the exercises in one session, or just a few at a time. Remember that your movements should be slow and soft, and they should not cause fatigue.

SET 1 ▍ Grasping and scratching

1 **Do this exercise immediately after you wake up in the morning. You can stay in** bed and just throw off the covers. Lie on your back with your legs stretched out, your arms at your sides.

2 **Perform grasping and scratching motions with your hands and feet 50** to 100 times.

ESSENTIAL POINTS

■ Relax your body and just let the ground support you.

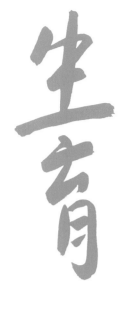

1

2

SET 2 ▮ Arm and leg rolls

1 **Lie on your back with your legs slightly apart** and your arms comfortably alongside your body, with the palms facing up.

2 Roll your arms over, so that the palms are now facing down.

3 Roll your arms farther toward the body, then back to the starting position. Repeat this action 50 times.

4 Next roll your legs inward, so that the feet are facing each other.

5 Roll the legs outward, so that the feet are now facing in opposite directions. Repeat 50 to 100 times.

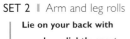

SET 3 | Pelvic tilts

| Lie on your back with your legs straight out and
together. Bend your knees and draw your feet up
to your buttocks.

1a

1b

2 Lift your pelvis while
constricting your anus.
Then lower your pelvis
slowly and relax your anus.

2a

2b

3 With your hips back on the
bed or floor, face the soles of
your feet toward each other and
slowly relax your thigh muscles
so that your knees spread as
wide as possible. Breathe in
and out deeply 3 times.
Then extend your
legs to their full
length. Repeat
this exercise
10 to 20 times.

3

SET 4 | Opposite hand touching

1 **Lie on your back in the shape of a cross —with your feet together and your arms** straight out to the sides.

2 **Trying to keep your hips still, reach across your body with your right hand** toward the left, which should not move. Turn to the other side and reach across your body with your left hand toward your right. Try to touch each hand 10 or more times.

ARMS ARE
OUTSTRETCHED

2

1

SET 5 | Muscle tensing and relaxing

1 | Lie on your back with your legs naturally extended.

2 Tense and relax your anal and vulval muscles 30 to 50 times. (To tense your anal muscles, imagine trying to stop a bowel movement; to tense your vulval muscles, imagine trying to stop urinating mid-flow.) Try to coordinate this exercise with your breathing rhythm —inhale while tensing and exhale while relaxing.

ESSENTIAL POINTS

- Move your body slowly and gently.
- There should be no unnecessary stress.

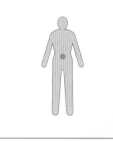

SET 6 Lunges

1 | Stand with your hands on your hips and take a long step forward with your right leg to form an arch. Your weight should be on your right leg, which is bent, and your left leg should be straight.

2 Then step forward onto your left leg, transferring your weight to it. Repeat 4 to 8 times with each leg.

● *In the last trimester, from the seventh month of pregnancy to the time of delivery, the body weight of the expectant mother increases so much that the center of gravity shifts toward the front. Because it is difficult to maintain balance during this stage, she should concentrate on exercises that are performed on her back. To avoid fatigue, the amount of exercise may be reduced, particularly during the last month of pregnancy.*

SET 7 ▮ Knee lifts

1 **Stand with your feet shoulder-width apart and your hands on your hips. Lift your right knee as high as you can,**

2 **Now lift the left leg. Keep your back straight and lift the knees one after the other. Do this 4 to 8 times per knee. If it is difficult to keep your balance, you can hold onto something, such as a chair back, for support.**

SET 8 ▮ Foot circling

1 **Stand on your left leg and raise your right foot off the ground.**

2 **Turn it around in circles, fully stretching the ankle. Do the same with the left foot. Repeat the sequence 4 to 8 times. If it is difficult to keep your balance, you can hold onto something, such as a chair back, for support.**

SET 9 ▮ Heel lifts

Stand with your feet shoulder-width apart and your hands on your hips. Without bending your knee, lift your left heel off the ground. Alternate with the other heel. Do this 4 to 8 times for each foot. If it is difficult to keep your balance, you can hold onto something, such as a chair back, for support.

LEFT HEEL IS RAISED SLIGHTLY OFF THE GROUND

100%

100%

75%

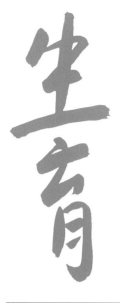

(44)

CHAN HOU FU WAN ZHI YUN DONG

Healing Exercises for After the Baby

The process of childbirth takes its toll on a woman's resources. After the birth, the new mother may feel tired and weak for some time. Her stomach and her intestines will not be functioning as well as they should, and the muscles of her pelvic floor and abdominal region will be slack.

Therapeutic exercises after childbirth can shorten the time required for recuperation. They strengthen both abdominal and pelvic floor muscles and speed up the return of the uterus to its pre-pregnancy state. They also help restore the normal workings of the stomach and intestines.

ESSENTIAL POINTS

■ Regaining lower-body muscle tone will help the health of the overall body.

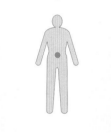

SET 2 ▌ Bent-knee leg raises

1 Lie on your back with your arms resting comfortably at your sides.

2 Raise one leg with the knee bent, then lower it.

3 Alternate with the other leg. Repeat several times.

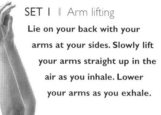

SET 1 ▌ Arm lifting
Lie on your back with your arms at your sides. Slowly lift your arms straight up in the air as you inhale. Lower your arms as you exhale.

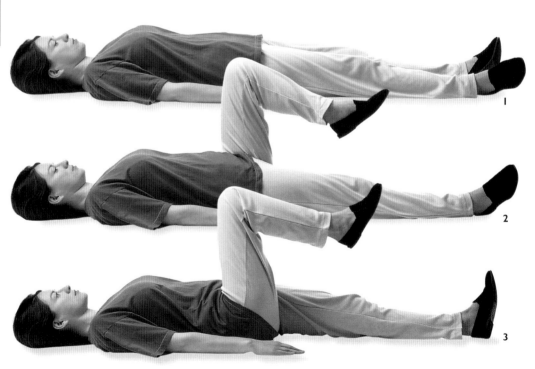

Generally, if the delivery has gone smoothly, then the new mother can begin to exercise 12 to 16 hours after childbirth.

Two groups of exercises follow on these and the next two pages. You can do whichever you like. In the beginning, repeat each exercise 4 to 6 times. Later on, increase to 8 to 12 repetitions. You can increase or decrease the number of repetitions depending on your strength and recovery. This will also affect the number of times you do the exercises each day.

Arm lifting, bent-knee leg raises, and hip raises can be performed the day after delivery. On the third day you can add sideways leg raises to these three; on the fourth day you can add heel raises and bent-knee sit-ups. From the fifth to seventh days, you can perform the entire group.

SET 2 ▮ Hip raises

1 Lie on your back with your knees bent, your feet flat on the bed and your arms resting by your side.

2 Lift your hips from the bed, then lower them.

SET 3 ▮ Sideways leg raises

Lie on your right side, with your right arm under your head. Bend and lift your left leg, then lower it. You can use your left hand for support if necessary. Repeat and then turn over and do the exercise with the other leg.

SET 4 ▮ Bent-knee sit-ups

1 Lie on your back with your knees bent.

2 Raise your head and do sit-ups. If this is difficult at first, you can use your arms for support. Later do the sit-up exercise without holding on to anything.

SET 5 ▮ Cycling

Lie on your back and lift your legs in the air. Pretend to ride a bicycle as you extend and bend your legs in turn.

SET 6 ❚ Grasping and scratching

1 **Lie on your back with your legs naturally stretched out and your arms at your sides.**

2 **Slowly perform grasping and scratching motions with your hands and feet 50 to 100 times.**

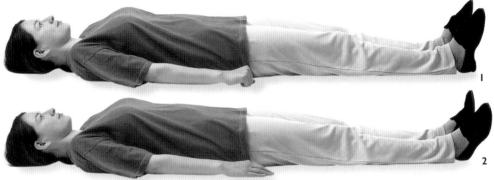

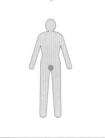

ESSENTIAL POINTS

■ Relax and let the ground support you.

■ Concentrate on the area that is being exercised.

SET 7 ❚ Anus constriction

Lie on your back with your legs naturally extended and your arms at your sides. Constrict your anus—imagine you are trying to stop a bowel movement—as you breathe in. Relax your anus as you breathe out. Repeat 5 to 7 times.

SET 8 ❚ Foot slides

1 **Lie on your back with your legs stretched out and your arms at your sides. Bend your knees and draw your heels toward your buttocks as you breathe in deeply.**

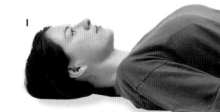

2 **As you breathe out deeply, let your feet slide back down until your legs are fully extended again. Repeat 3 to 7 times.**

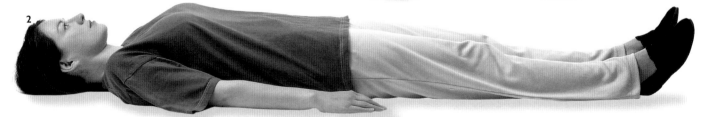

SET 9 | Hip raises

1 Lie on your back with your knees bent and your heels as close to your buttocks as possible. Place your hands under your head.

2 Lift your hips off the bed as you breathe in deeply. Your weight should be on your shoulders and the soles of your feet. Breathe out deeply as you lower your hips.

3 Then constrict your anus while breathing in and relax it while breathing out. Repeat the whole exercise 3 to 7 times.

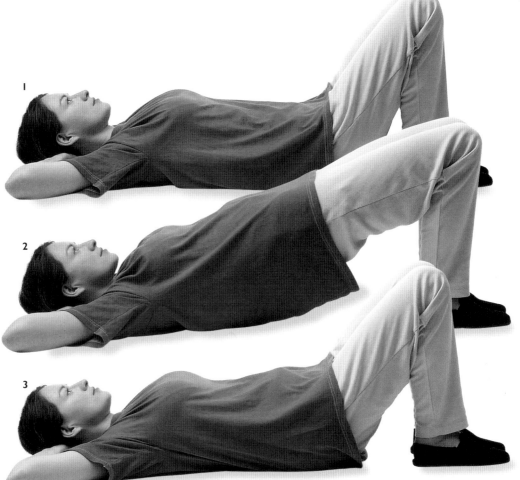

SET 10 | Arm stretching

1 Lie on your back with your arms at your sides. Draw your hands up along your sides, bending your elbows. Continue raising your hands across your shoulders and up behind your head as you inhale.

2 Exhale as you draw your arms back down. Repeat 3 to 7 times.

生育

45

KANG FU YUN DONG HE TENG DONG JIE DUAN

Healing Exercises for Painful Periods

Dysmenorrhea is pain that occurs just before or at the onset of menstruation. The pain, which may be cramplike, is centered in the lower abdomen. There are two types. Primary dysmenorrhea affects young women having their first periods. Psychological factors, weak abdominal muscles, and an underdeveloped or misplaced uterus may all play a role. Secondary dysmenorrhea is caused by gynecological disorders such as an inflammation of the reproductive organs.

Therapeutic exercise works better for primary dysmenorrhea than for secondary. It can improve blood circulation in the pelvic cavity, strengthen abdominal muscles, and contribute to an improved mental state. Do the following exercises 2 or 3 times a day before or at the onset of menstruation.

ESSENTIAL POINTS

■ Gentle lower abdominal breathing while sitting or standing is also good for dysmenorrhea.

SET 1 | Heel lifts

1 **Stand with your feet shoulder-width apart and hold onto the back of a chair. Without bending your legs, lift and lower the right heel.**

2 **Lift and lower the other heel. Do this 20 times.**

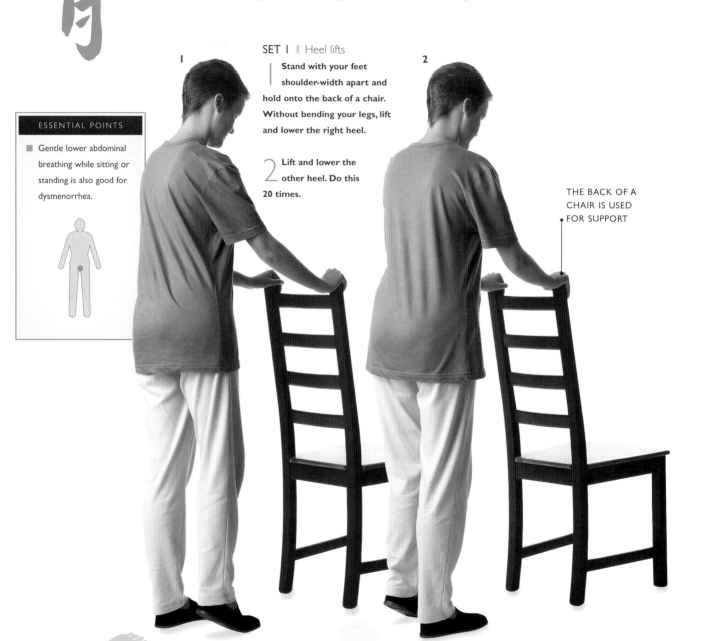

1

2

THE BACK OF A CHAIR IS USED FOR SUPPORT

75%

75%

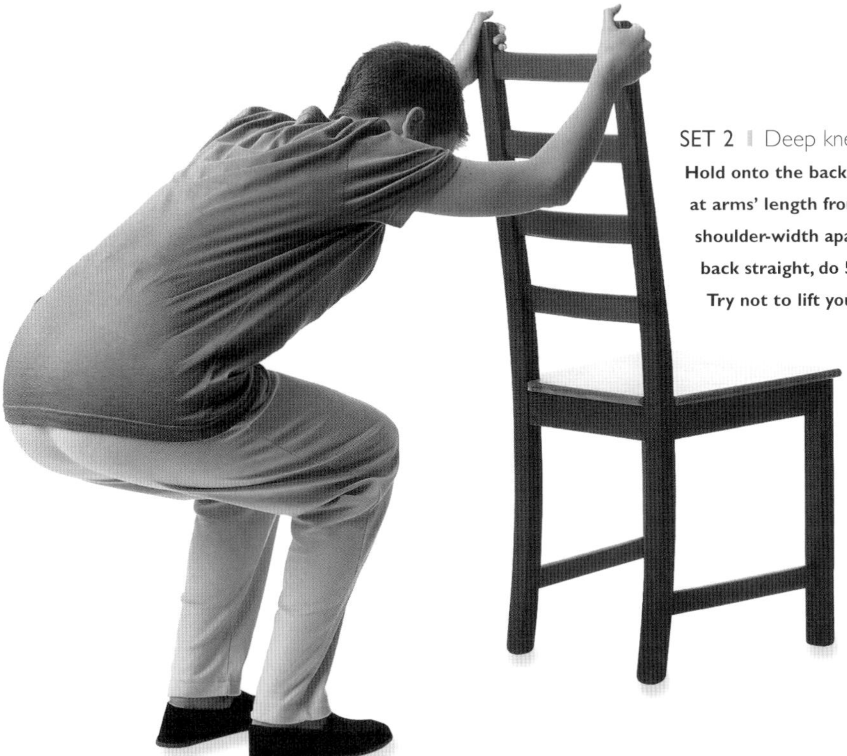

SET 2 ‖ Deep knee bends

Hold onto the back of a chair and stand at arms' length from it, with your feet shoulder-width apart. Keeping your back straight, do 5 deep knee bends. Try not to lift your heels off the floor.

SET 3 ‖ Abdominal breathing

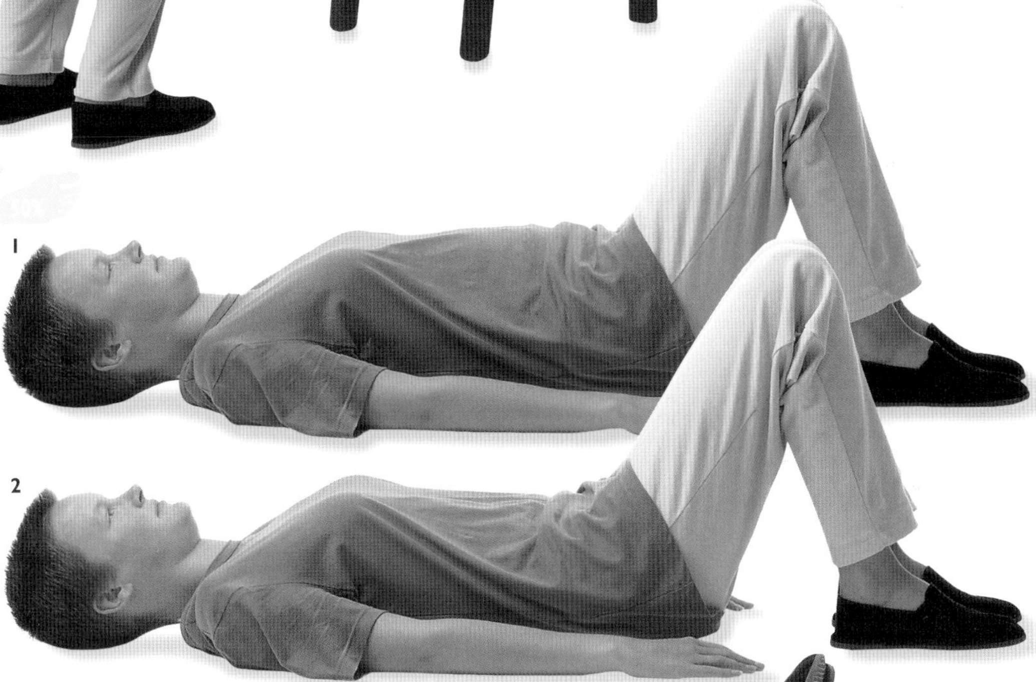

| Lie on your back with your legs bent and knees raised. **Perform abdominal breathing about 10 times. Feel your abdomen slowly inflate like a balloon as you breathe in through your nose,**

2 **Then feel the abdomen slowly fall as you breathe out through your mouth. You** can rest your hands lightly on your abdomen if you like, so that you can feel the movement in it.

SET 4 ‖ Knee raises

Lie on your back with your arms at your sides. Lift your knees and bring them up to touch your chin, supporting your lower back with your hands. Repeat about 10 times.

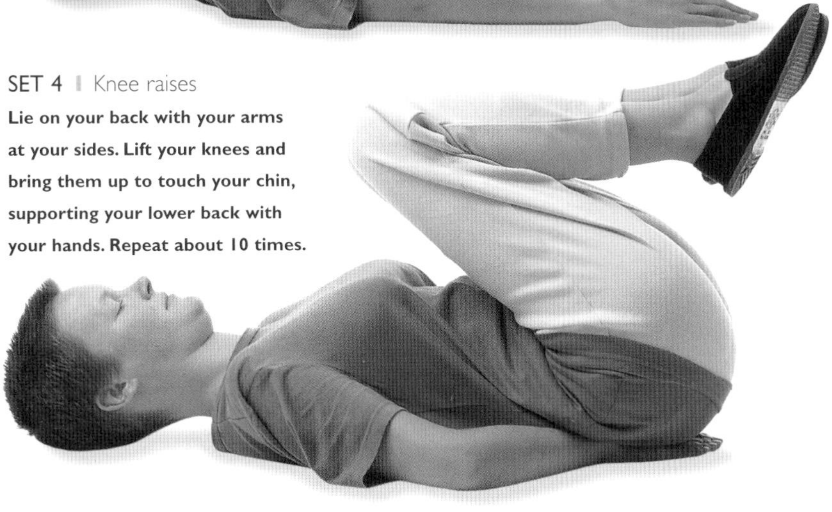

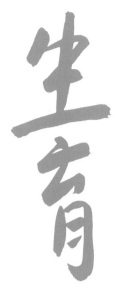

(46)

PAN GU DE JI ROU

The Muscles of the Pelvic Floor

The muscles of the pelvic floor, also known as the pelvic diaphragm, collectively make up the levator ani muscle, which includes the pubococcygeus, iliococcygeus, and sacrococcygeal muscles. The pubococcygeus muscle is the largest and strongest, interlaces with the sphincter muscle of the urethra—the outlet of the tube that leads from the bladder—and inserts into the vaginal sphincter, a circle-shaped contracting muscle.

The levator ani muscle has two important functions. It supports the organs situated inside the pelvic cavity and it constricts the lower end of the rectum and the vagina. It is also closely related to the sphincter muscles of the urinary bladder and the urethra. The muscles of the pelvic floor are frequently blamed whenever urinary incontinence occurs.

Do each of the following exercises several times, until you feel mildly fatigued. The first exercise is the most important—you can do it on its own and still expect good results. Practice it 2 or 3 times a day for 15 to 20 minutes at a time, or do it 200 times in a row.

ESSENTIAL POINTS

■ Both men and women gain health benefits from pelvic-floor exercises.

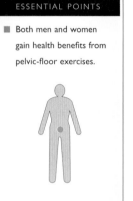

SET I ▍ Pelvic-muscle contraction

1 **Lie on your back. Breathe in, lift your hips slightly, and contract the muscles of the pelvic floor—it should feel like trying to hold back a bowel movement.**

2 **Breathe out as you relax the muscles of the pelvic floor and loosen your body.**

1

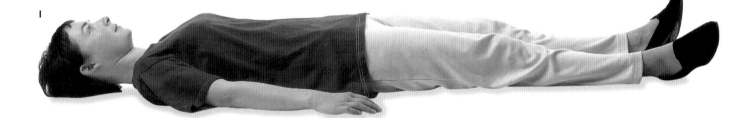

2

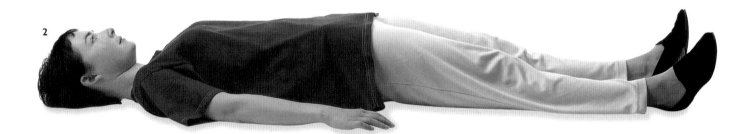

SET 2 | Lower back lift

1 | Lie on your back with your knees bent. Breathe in and lift the sacral region—your lower back—contracting your buttocks, hip, and pelvic-floor muscles as you do so.

2 Let go slowly and lower yourself back onto the ground. Relax your entire body.

SET 3 | Crossed-ankle lift

1 | Lie on your back with your legs full length but crossed at the ankles. Place your feet against a wall.

2 While breathing in, tighten the muscles of the pelvic floor and lift just your lower back from the bed.

3 Next, lift both your head and your hips slightly while you breathe in.

4 Relax your entire body as you breathe out.

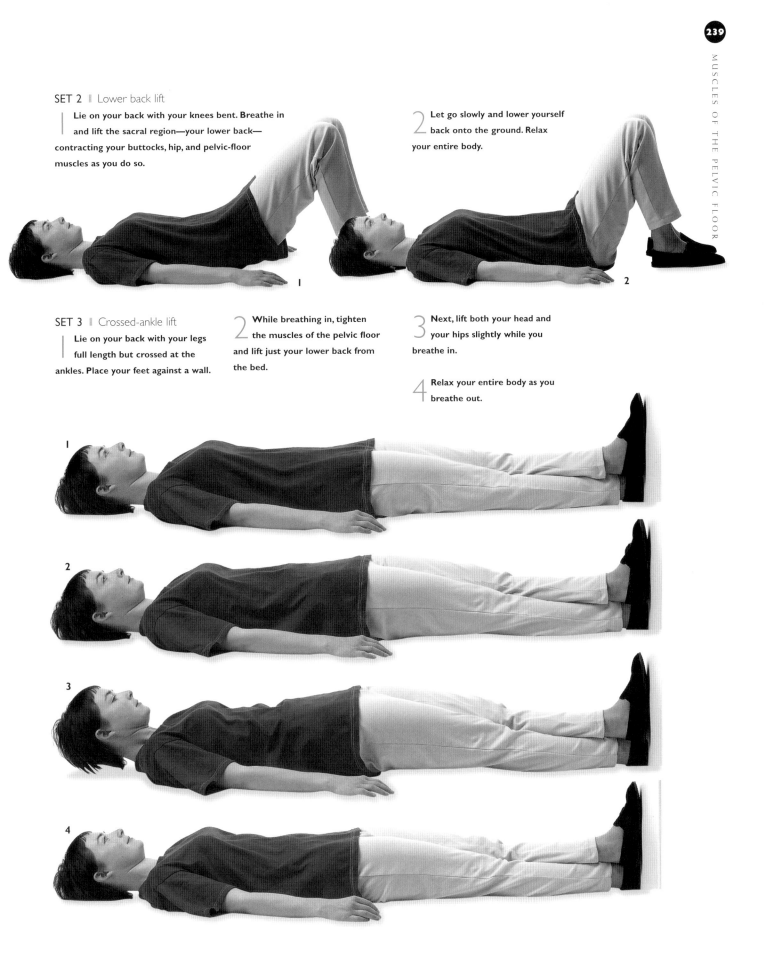

SET 4 | Knee squeeze

1 | Lie on your back with your legs drawn up to your body and knees bent.

2 Press your knees against each other as hard as possible while simultaneously raising your pelvis.

3 Then relax your thighs and lower your pelvis back to the ground.

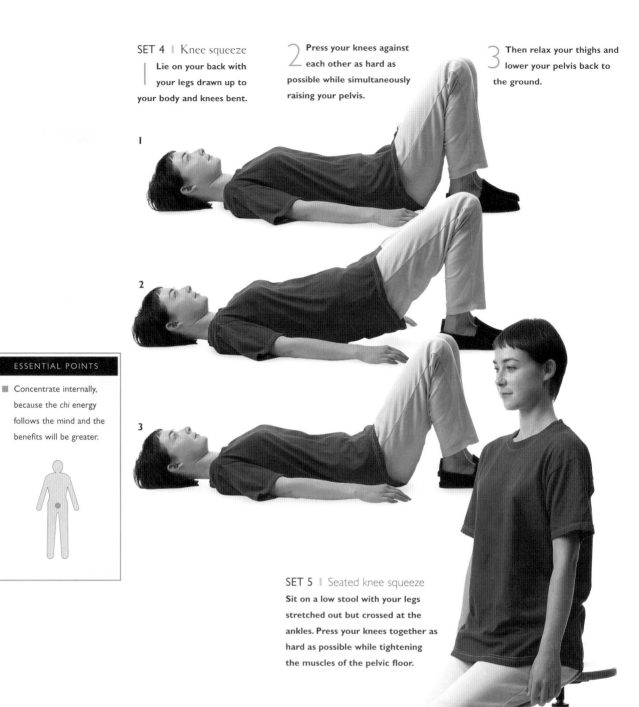

1

2

ESSENTIAL POINTS

■ Concentrate internally, because the *chi* energy follows the mind and the benefits will be greater.

3

SET 5 | Seated knee squeeze

Sit on a low stool with your legs stretched out but crossed at the ankles. Press your knees together as hard as possible while tightening the muscles of the pelvic floor.

SET 6 ▌ Back curve

1 **Kneel on your hands and knees. Arch** your lumbar vertebrae—the mid-back—in a raised curve and contract the muscles of the pelvic floor as you breathe in.

2 **Relax your back as you breathe out.**

Squatting contraction

1 **Squat with your buttocks resting on your heels.**

2 **As you inhale, tighten your hip, buttocks, and** pelvic floor muscles, then lean forward and put your hands on the floor, assuming a kneeling position.

3 **Return to the squat and relax your muscles as you** breathe out.

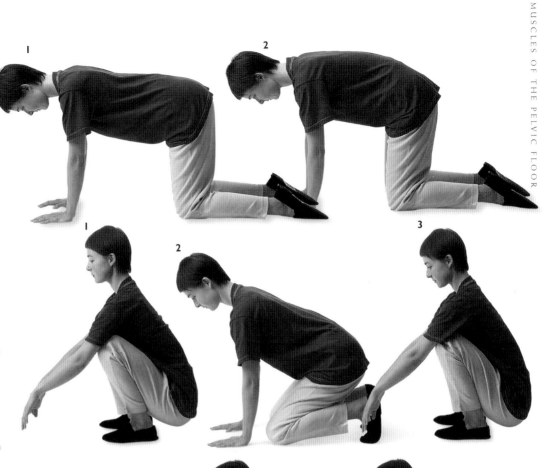

SET 8 ▌ Seated contraction

1 **Sit on a high stool. Lifting your feet from the floor, contract** the muscles in your pelvic floor as you breathe in.

2 **Relax the pelvic muscles and lower your feet as you breathe** out again.

生育

(47)

ZHI LIAO PANG GUANG YAN

Healing Cystitis

Cystitis is the most common bladder disorder. Its symptoms include frequent and painful urination and the passing of pus or blood in the urine. In chronic cystitis, the inflammation may affect part or all of the mucous membrane; sometimes the symptoms are mild and may even be overlooked. However, chronic cystitis is a stubborn disease that resists treatment, although healing exercise can help relieve it.

Do each of the following exercises as many times as feels comfortable, unless directed otherwise.

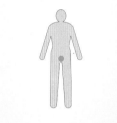

ESSENTIAL POINTS

■ Chinese herbal medicine is also quite effective in treating cystitis.

SET 1 | Foot turning

1 Lie on your back with your legs extended and about 24in (60cm) apart. Turn your feet out.

2 Turn your feet in to face each other, causing your legs to roll slightly from side to side.

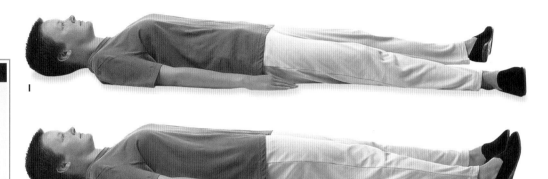

SET 2 | Hip raises

1 Lie on your back with your knees bent and your feet close to your buttocks. Raise your hips as high into the air as possible as you breathe in deeply.

2 Lower your hips as you breathe out.

SET 3 | Cycling

Lie on your back and lift your legs in the air. Ride an imaginary bicycle, as you alternately extend and bend your legs.

CAUTION

People with acute cystitis—the severe, active form of the disease—should not exercise. They should see a doctor and take plenty of rest.

SET 4 | Leg crossing and circling

1 Lie on your back with your legs straight up. Cross your legs back and forth over each other in a sideways scissors motion.

2 With your legs still crossed, draw small circles in the air.

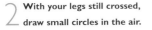

1

2

SET 5 | Massage

1 Stand with your back straight and your feet shoulder-width apart. Rub and push on the area around your coccyx (tailbone) with both hands for a few minutes. Knock this area hard 30 or more times with one fist.

2 Then stand with your legs together, breathe in deeply and squat down as low as you can.

3 Wrap your arms around your knees and squeeze as you breathe out fully. Repeat 6 to 7 times. If you want more of a workout, you can do the exercises for silicosis patients (*see pp. 144–145*).

1a

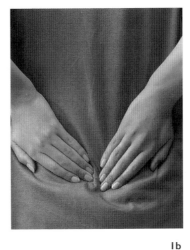

1b

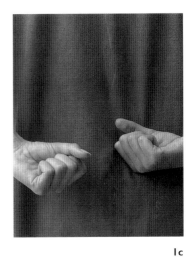

1c

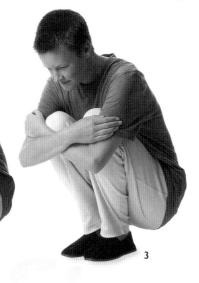

2

3

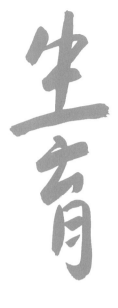

(48)

SHI GE QIAN LIE XIAN HE JING NANG YAN BING REN DE YUN DONG

Exercises for Prostatitis and Vesiculitis

Patients with chronic prostatitis, an inflammation of the prostate gland, tend also to suffer from chronic vesiculitis, inflammation of the seminal vesicles. Some men do not even notice the symptoms of these diseases, but others are more sensitive to them. Some experience pain, usually in their lower back, buttocks, pelvic floor, groin, or sex organs. They may also feel it in their lower abdomen and legs. If the inflammation is long-standing, the patient may also suffer headaches and dizziness. If the condition gets worse, he may not be able to sit for long because of the pain in the lower back and pelvic areas.

Prostatitis may also cause frequent and painful urination and a feeling that the bladder is not empty. The urethra may sting and burn, or there may be white secretions coming from it. These are signs of an inflamed prostate and typically

ESSENTIAL POINTS

■ Chinese herbal medicine is effective in treating prostatitis and vesiculitis.

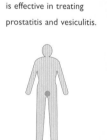

SET 1 ▮ Chinese "buttock-vibrating" exercise

1 Lie on your back with your legs naturally extended and your arms by your side.

2 Alternately tighten and relax your buttocks as fast as you can so that your hips jiggle up and down. Repeat this until your muscles are tired. The aim of the exercise is to loosen your pelvis and get the energy moving there.

1

2

SET 2 ▮ Hip raises

1 Lie on your back with your legs drawn up and your feet near your buttocks. Using your shoulders and feet for support, lift your hips high off the bed, constrict your anus and breathe in deeply.

2 Then let go suddenly and let your hips drop to the bed to vibrate your pelvic area. As your hips fall, relax your entire body and breathe out deeply. Repeat this 10 to 20 times.

1

2

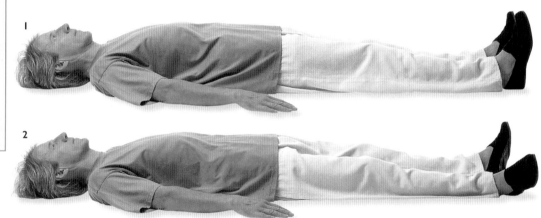

appear when the patient gets out of bed or after he has a bowel movement. Premature ejaculation, impotence, a loss of sexual desire, and nocturnal emissions may also occur.

No totally satisfactory treatment of chronic prostatitis and vesiculitis has yet been found. In recent years, the use of a comprehensive approach, combining traditional Chinese medicine with Western medicine, therapeutic exercises, and warm-water baths of 10 to 20 minutes each night has proved helpful in alleviating the symptoms. In addition to the following exercises, both Tai Chi (*see pp. 60–67*) and Nei Yang Kung, internally nourishing breathing (*see pp. 78–79*), have proved effective.

SET 3 | Goldfish exercise

1 **Lie on your back with your legs naturally extended and your hands behind your head.**

2 **Sway your waist from side to side like a fish swimming. Repeat 100 to 200 times. You may also** do the same exercise on your stomach, which is especially effective for treating constipation and abdominal bloating.

SET 4 | "Fanning" exercise

1 **Lie on your back, lift your legs 40 to 50 degrees off the bed.**

2 **Cross your legs 50 to 100 times, rather like a Chinese paper fan opening and closing.**

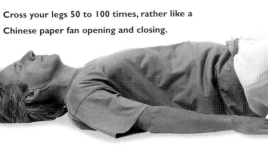

SET 5 ▌ Cycling

Lie on your back, raise your feet in the air and pedal as if you were riding a bicycle. Do this at least 50 to 100 times.

SET 6 ▌ Kidney- and waist-strengthening exercise

1 **This is a self-massage combined with a stretch. Stand with your feet slightly more than shoulder-width apart. Rub around your navel with both hands.**

2 **Continue rubbing around the sides of your waist to the small of your back and your tailbone.**

3 **Bend forward and massage down the outer sides of your legs, around your feet, and up the insides of your legs until your hands are back at the starting point near your navel. Repeat the sequence 20 to 30 times.**

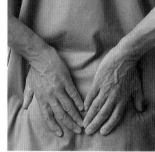

2b

ESSENTIAL POINTS

■ The healing energy of the body follows the mind, so concentrating internally will bring results.

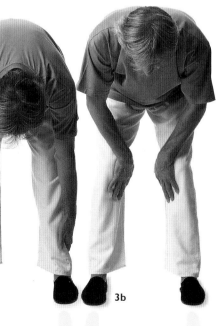

1   2a   3a   3b

SET 7 | Knocking at the gate

1 Stand naturally with your feet shoulder-width apart and make loose fists with your hands. Turn your body from side to side, using the small of your back as the axis. As you turn to the left, knock your lower abdomen with your right fist,

2 At the same time knock your tailbone with your left hand. Change hands and repeat as often as you like.

SET 8 | Brick-lifting exercise

1 First prepare a relatively simple piece of equipment. Find a wooden rod that is 1½–2in (3.75–5cm) thick and as long as your shoulders are wide. Drill a hole through the middle of the rod. Tie one end of a piece of string firmly to the rod through the hole and tie the other end to a brick or a can weighing no more than 5lb (2.25kg). To begin the exercise, stand as if you were riding a horse, legs wide apart, knees bent and toes firmly clutching the ground. Hold the rod horizontally in front of you, one hand on each end and your tigers' mouths—the space between your thumbs and index fingers—facing each other.

2 Now use your hands to roll the string up until the brick or can is at chest level. Release the string and lower the object slowly. Repeat several times. The weight of the brick and the number of times you perform this can be increased gradually.

3 Then knock or strike your arms, chest, and abdomen with loose fists or palms to give yourself a massage and stimulate your circulation.

1

2

1

2a

2b

生育

Healing Exercises to Improve Varicocele

Varicocele—varicose veins located in the network that lies along the spermatic cord—occurs most frequently on the left side of the body, in 20- to 30-year-old men, but like many conditions it may be helped by healing exercises, which will strengthen the abdominal muscles and improve circulation of the blood in the pelvic cavity.

In most cases, this condition is not even noticed until it is discovered during a medical examination. Varicocele rarely needs special medical treatment unless it impairs sperm production or causes swelling, pain, or a feeling of downward displacement. The condition may improve on its own in some young patients after they marry.

In cases of varicocele it is recommended that patients move their bowels regularly and avoid chronic constipation by consuming plenty of whole grains, fresh fruit and vegetables, and water.

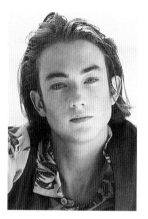

■ **Varicocele is most common in young men, but often goes unnoticed for some time.**

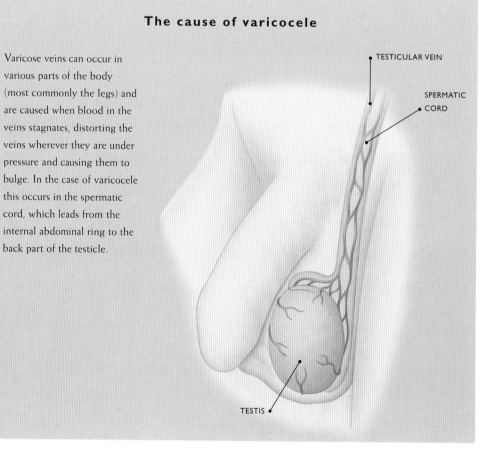

The cause of varicocele

Varicose veins can occur in various parts of the body (most commonly the legs) and are caused when blood in the veins stagnates, distorting the veins wherever they are under pressure and causing them to bulge. In the case of varicocele this occurs in the spermatic cord, which leads from the internal abdominal ring to the back part of the testicle.

TESTICULAR VEIN

SPERMATIC CORD

TESTIS

To alleviate symptoms, try taking a cold bath or washing the area with cold water, which will cause the spermatic veins to constrict and reduce blood congestion in the veins. The best healing exercises are those designed to strengthen the muscles in the abdominal walls and to facilitate blood circulation in the pelvic cavity. The exercises to strengthen the muscles of the pelvic floor (*see pp. 238–241*) can help, as can those for dealing with habitual constipation (*see pp. 150–153*). By moving his bowels regularly and avoiding constipation, a man will minimize the chance of waste matter increasing pressure on the left spermatic veins, thus hindering the return of blood to the heart.

■ Pushing and pressing down on the abdomen, with one hand on top of the other, may help.

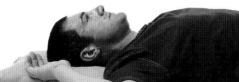

■ Pretending to pedal a bicycle can help to alleviate constipation, a contributory factor.

■ Deep abdominal breathing can strengthen the muscles of the abdomen.

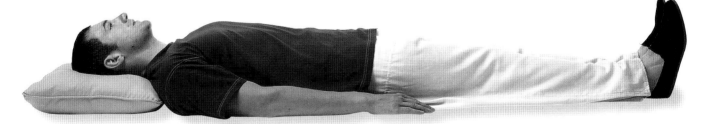

Glossary

Abdomen: The area of the body that lies between the pelvis and the chest.

Abdominal breathing: A form of breathing technique that involves long, slow, deep inhalation and exhalation; it is dependent on contraction between the abdominal muscles and diaphragm.

Acupuncture points: Points situated on the body where the flow of energy or *chi* through the body may be adjusted.

An Mu: Chinese massage, which uses principally the techniques of knocking, beating, and patting, rather than the kneading and rubbing more common in Western massage.

Arrhythmia: An irregularity in the rhythm of the heart, usually a premature contraction.

Arteriosclerosis: Hardening of the arteries, caused by a build-up of fats in the blood.

Asthma: Narrowing of the bronchial airways, causing wheezing and coughing.

Bubbling Spring: *See* Yung Chuan.

Buerger's Disease: A circulatory disorder of the arteries and veins; also known as Thromboangitis obliterans.

Chi: Natural healing energy, the universal life force.

Chiang Chuang Kung: Invigorating breathing, which pays special attention to *ju ching*; less demanding than some types of Chi Kung, so useful for those who are physically weak.

Chien Ming Men: *See* Tan Tien.

Chi Kung: Self-healing exercises, or The Art of Breathing; it combines mental concentration with breathing exercises.

Ching Ming: An acupuncture point located just beyond the inner corner of the eye; used to treat eye conditions.

Chronic bronchitis: A condition that causes inflammation and narrowing of the air passages, resulting in breathing difficulties.

Chronic obstructive pulmonary disease: Covers a range of lung disorders that cause difficulty in breathing, most commonly emphysema and chronic bronchitis.

Coronary artery disease: Thickening of the walls of the vessels that supply the heart, thus reducing the flow of blood.

Dysmenorrhea: Pain just before or at the start of menstruation.

Eight Sets of Embroidery, The: Exercises to increase arm and leg strength and develop the chest; they may be performed with or without force.

Emphysema: A degenerative disease of the lungs, which causes breathlessness.

Fang Sung Kung: Relaxation breathing, whereby the whole body is gradually relaxed by means of *ju ching*.

Feng Chih: An acupuncture point located on each side of the neck; also known as Windy Lake. Used to bring relief from colds.

Five Animal Play: Ancient Chinese exercises that mimic the gestures of the tiger, deer, bear, monkey, and bird.

Ha Ku: An acupuncture point on the index finger, located just beside the first joint; used to treat abdominal pain.

Hand swinging: *See* Li Shou.

Hau Ming Men: *See* Ming Men.

Hemorrhoids: Varicose veins in the soft lining of the anus; also called piles.

Hypertension: High blood pressure.

Invigorating breathing: *See* Chiang Chuang Kung.

Kidney 1: *See* Yung Chuan.

Knocking at the Gate of Life: The ancient fitness technique that combines massage, knocking, and waist exercise; the Chinese term Tsa Fu Pei means literally to knock the abdomen and back.

Kung fu: Mastery of a mental or physical feat through regular practice.

Ju ching: The state of entering into mental quietness using words that induce relaxation, such as "quiet" and "relax."

Li Shou: Hand swinging movements, designed to build up strength and resistance to disease.

Lordosis: The medical name for the condition hollow back or saddleback, in which the spine curves toward the front.

Meridian: An energy channel or pathway along which vital energy (*chi*) flows to the body's organs. There are 12 main meridians and other, lesser meridians.

Ming Men: The position on the back (Life Gate) that corresponds to Tan Tien on the front of the body; also known as Hau Ming Men (The Back Gate of Life).

Neijing: *See* Yellow Emperor.

Nei Yang Kung: Internally nourishing breathing, which pays particular attention to the actual technique of breathing.

Organ: In TCM there are 12 main organs of the body, corresponding to the 12 main meridians: the Lungs, Liver, Gall

Bladder, Large Intestine, Bladder, Small Intestine, Spleen, Stomach, Kidneys, Heart, Pericardium, and Triple Heater.

Pace-determined walking program: A form of therapy that involves walking at a set pace over a specific distance, which is gradually increased and timed.

Pai-Hui: An acupuncture point located in the exact middle of the flat part at the top of the head; used to treat gray hair.

Pa Tuan Chin: *See* Eight Sets of Embroidery.

Pericardium: The outer, protective layers of the heart.

Prostatitis: Inflammation of the prostate gland.

Purpura: A bleeding disease that creates purplish or reddish blotches on the skin as the blood leeches into it.

Rectal prolapse: A condition whereby mucous membranes become detached from the rectum and then protrude from the anus.

Relaxation breathing: *See* Fang Sung Kung.

Respectable Kidney: *See* Shen Yu.

Sciatica: A nerve condition causing severe pain in the buttocks and down one leg.

Scoliosis: A condition in which there is curvature of the spine; there are two types: sickle- or C-shaped; and snake- or S-shaped.

Shen Yu: An acupuncture point in the small of the back, over the kidneys; also known as Respectable Kidney.

Shih Erh Tuan Chin: *See* Twelve Sets of Embroidery.

Shun San: An acupuncture point located on the leg that may be used to treat abdominal pain.

Silicosis: A form of lung disease caused by inhaling silica.

Ssu-Pai: An acupuncture point located on the side of the bridge of the nose; used to treat eye conditions.

Tai Chi Chuan: Yin-Yang Boxing, originally a form of martial art, but now more generally associated with self-healing; often abbreviated to Tai Chi.

Tai Chi Rod/Ruler: Tai Chi exercises that use a rod or ruler, made of wood and about 12in (30cm) long.

Tai Yang: An acupuncture point located in the hollow just below the end of the eyebrow; used to treat eye conditions.

Tan Tien: The important area in TCM that is located 3in (7.5cm) below the navel; also called Chien Ming Men (The Front Gate of Life); means literally "Field of the Elixir."

Therapeutic gymnastics: Gymnastic exercises that are designed to help heal specific diseases.

Thromboangitis obliterans: *See* Buerger's Disease.

Tien Yin: An acupuncture point situated between the eyebrow and upper corner of the orbital cavity; used to treat eye conditions.

Traditional Chinese medicine (TCM): The system of Chinese medicine that has been practiced in China for nearly 5000 years.

Triple Heater: The organ in TCM that controls the distribution of Heat and Water; sometimes known as the San Jiao.

Tsa Fu Pei: *See* Knocking at the Gate of Life.

Tsu San Li: An acupuncture point located on the leg that may be used to treat abdominal pain.

Twelve Sets of Embroidery, The: Exercises made up of self-massage and fitness movements.

Varicocele: The condition when varicose veins occur in the network that lies along the spermatic cord.

Vesiculitis: Inflammation of the seminal vesicles.

Wei Chuan: An acupuncture point located on the leg that may be used to treat abdominal pain.

Welcome Fragrance: *See* Yin Shen.

Windy Lake: *See* Feng Chih.

Yang: In Chinese philosophy, Yang is one aspect of the complementary opposites—Yin being the other aspect; it is associated with warmth, activity, and brightness.

Yee Chin Ching: Exercises that develop the muscles and tendons.

Yellow Emperor: Author of the formative TCM work, the *Neijing* ("The Classic of Internal Medicine").

Yin: The opposite aspect in Chinese philosophy to Yang; it is associated with coldness, passivity, and dampness.

Yin Shen: An acupuncture point on the side of the nose, near the flare of the nostrils; also known as Welcome Fragrance; used to treat nasal congestion.

Yuen chi: The ability of the body to resist disease, adapt to the environment that surrounds it and restore proper internal functioning.

Yung Chuan: The acupuncture point located one-third of the way down the foot, in the depression made when the toes are curled under; also known as Bubbling Spring or Kidney 1. It forms the starting point of the Foot-Lesser Yin-Kidney Meridian.

Index

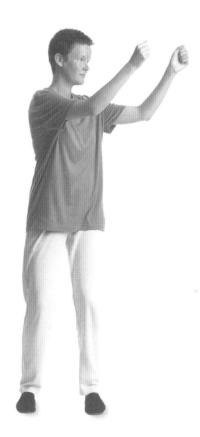

Acknowledgments

Picture credits

All pictures by Guy Ryecart except the following:

e. t. archive: p26

The Hutchison Library: pps2 (Melanie Friend), 8ML (Felix Greene), 11 (John Hatt), 14ML (Michael Macintyre), 104ML (Jeremy Horner), 148M (Aymon Frank)

The Image Bank, London: pps12ML, 96B, 97TR, 110, 122M, 123, 124B, 125TL, 127B, 131M, 169T, 174M, 225T, 248

Images Colour Library: pps10M, 17T

Tony Stone/Getty Images, London: pps16, 18R, 19, 23T, 24M, 25, 36, 68L, 94M, 95, 98 (both), 102ML, 104B, 106ML, 108ML and B, 109R, 162M, 163T, 165BL, 165T, 175, 185, 222, 223

Other credits

The publishers would like to thank: Guy Ryecart for studio photography; Dina Christy for organizing the photoshoot; and Frankie Goldstone for prop hunting.

Many thanks also to Paul Brecher, for reading through the text, checking the photography, and advising on many parts of the book. Paul Brecher is a qualified Tai Chi instructor and practitioner of acupuncture who has written widely on the subject of Chinese medicine and healing exercise: for further information, see his website at **http://www.taiji.net**.

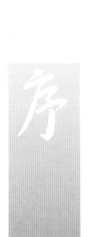

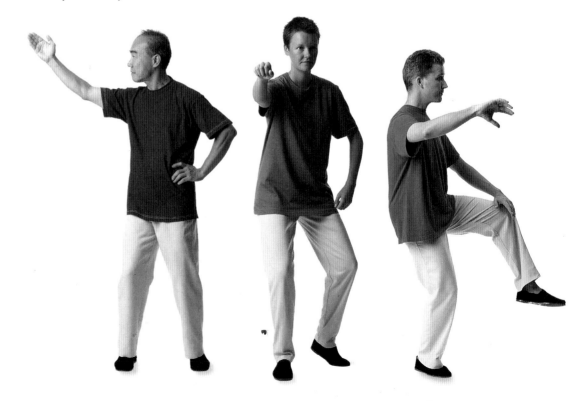